CARE

CARE

HOW PEOPLE OF FAITH

CAN RESPOND TO

OUR **BROKEN**

HEALTH SYSTEM

G. SCOTT MORRIS

WILLIAM B. EERDMANS PUBLISHING COMPANY
GRAND RAPIDS, MICHIGAN

Wm. B. Eerdmans Publishing Co.
4035 Park East Court SE, Grand Rapids, Michigan 49546
www.eerdmans.com

Published 2022
Printed in the United States of America

28 27 26 25 24 23 22   1 2 3 4 5 6 7

ISBN 978-0-8028-8237-0

Library of Congress Cataloging-in-Publication Data

A catalog record for this book is available from the Library of Congress.

Unless otherwise noted, Scripture quotations are from the New Revised Standard Version of the Bible.

To the staff, board, volunteers, and donors
who have helped Church Health thrive since 1987

CONTENTS

FOREWORD

I didn't know that John Wesley practiced medicine throughout his career. Wesley, the great English preacher, has been a mentor and model for me because he preached a holistic gospel—one that is both personal and social, transforming both lives and society. I once got to preach in Wesley's famous pulpit in London, and the feeling of being in a pulpit that changed the world was overwhelming for someone who believes that pulpits should change the world. Most don't. Wesley preferred traveling on horseback, reportedly over fifty thousand miles per year throughout the English countryside. In preaching the gospel, the founder of Methodism believed that healing the sick was central to the gospel message, as was caring for the poor. Both were essential to following after Jesus for John Wesley.

The author of this book, G. Scott Morris, MDiv and MD, is also a follower of Jesus in the tradition of Wesley, being an ordained Methodist minister and a practicing physician who opened Church Health in Memphis, Tennessee, thirty-five years ago because it was one of the poorest cities in the country. This book has a message and a mission—to show how the gospel of Jesus Christ is centrally and integrally connected to healing the sick and caring for the poor in both body and spirit. Scott Morris insists they cannot be separated. The gospel that changes lives and society always cares for the poor and heals the sick, which for Scott means the health care that leads to justice for those left out and left behind.

This is a wonderful book of stories: stories of the patients Scott has

treated with every kind of ailment and illness, especially health deficits
caused by the social determinants in the lives of the poorest Americans;
stories of the multitude of other faith-based health clinics that have sprung
up around the country; and stories of those called to serve the underserved
who are sick, because of their commitment to Jesus Christ. Some of the
best stories are the ones about the relationships between the medical doctors and nurses and the patients they meet and serve and how those relationships change everyone involved—as they should.

And throughout the book the story of the gospel shines. Jesus was God
made flesh—flesh and blood in a body who walked wherever he went in the
sun and rain, who got hungry and ate, who got tired and slept, who must
have felt better on some days than others. Jesus was fully God but also
fully human. He had to care for his own body, and he cared for the bodies
of others as central to his ministry. Jesus showed us how the whole person
relates to God and how to live a life of faith in a body.

I have never read a book so full of the stories of Jesus's healings, with
the texts of those healings woven through very human stories. Just Scott's
commentaries on Jesus's healings are worth the read, and the integration
of the gospel's healing texts and stories with the real-life stories of so many
people's health and healing is a wonderful combination that makes everything very real and very human.

I had heard some things about this but never realized how extensive and
extraordinary the response of Christians to the many and massive plagues
that ravaged Europe and the Roman world was to their very identity and
calling. It was Christians who were the ones who cared for the sick when
no one else would, even at risk to themselves. And when people recovered, they reportedly asked, "Who is your God, that I might worship him?"
Even the nonbelievers were impressed by how these Christians cared for
the poor and healed the sick. Wouldn't that be a wonderful thing were it
true today?

There is a remarkable chapter in this book about the COVID-19 pandemic. COVID-19 was revelatory, showing us the realities and inequities
of the world that we ignored, allowed, or just tolerated when we shouldn't
have. Scott Morris points those out with the realities that his clinic treated
during COVID-19. The poorest were clearly the first and hardest hit,
forced to bear the brunt of the suffering and death as "essential workers"

in constant contact with the virus and living in the most crowded house-holds as infections spread. And, of course, the overwhelming and dispro-portionate victims of COVID-19 were Black and Hispanic. Scott's chapter demonstrates the racialized story of COVID-19. The pandemic didn't dis-criminate—but we did. The greatest burden was borne by those who always bear the burdens of our inequities. Scott illustrates that what was true be-fore the pandemic became most visible during the pandemic, and it's un-likely to change after the pandemic unless we make the commitment not to return to "normal." He says, "COVID-19 cast a floodlight on the truth."

I was part of forming Faiths 4 Vaccines, the largest multifaith campaign to address the access and hesitancy issues around vaccinations. What we learned that worked was trusted locations and vocations to bring vaccina-tions to marginalized people. Clinics like Scott's were central to caring for the sick during the pandemic and revealed why and who became the sickest.

Healing the whole person, body and spirit, is the central theme of this book. And the most powerful accomplishment of this book is giving human faces to that healing—faces of the sick, faces of the poor, faces of the heal-ers, and faces of the system that has failed the poor. To my great delight, Scott includes a chapter that gives us the face of the woman who bolstered his inspiration to start his clinic. She is a special friend I first met years ago who demonstrates the face of Jesus more clearly, simply, and humbly than most Christians I have ever met on this planet. Dr. Janelle Goetcheus of Church of the Saviour in Washington, DC, became Jesus's doctor for the city's homeless and poor, walking the streets and the clinics with a cross around her neck. No matter what people believe about religion, no matter what their skepticism and cynicism, when people watch Janelle work and live, they think differently about what it means to be a Christian, just as so many people did when the first Christians cared for the poor and healed the sick in body and in spirit with the health that leads to justice.

Read this book about how to do that again.

Rev. Jim Wallis
Founder of Sojourners
Founding Director of Center on Faith and Justice

ONE

LIVING WATER IN CACTUS, TEXAS

"Two."

"You got drunk after two beers?" Dr. Stephanie Diehlmann was dubious. No one gets into a bar brawl and has his finger bitten after just two beers. And George was not a small man and was still young.

She cleaned George's red, swollen, tender, clearly infected finger and waited for the truth. Two beers before work. Two more during working hours. Two after work. That's what George grudgingly admitted to. Steph figured he drank at least twice what he confessed. George did some serious drinking all day every day.

Gently, Steph probed. "Do you get sick when you stop drinking?"

"I can't stop throwing up," George confided, "and I shake."

"Do you have nightmares?"

Instantly a thirty-two-year-old man, who was well over six feet tall and strong, began sobbing.

Now she was getting somewhere.

Initially, George was treated in an emergency room—not in Cactus because there isn't a hospital in the small town—a week earlier. He and a man he called his brother, meaning he was from the same tribe in South Sudan, had gotten into a fight while drunk, and the other man had bitten George's finger. The emergency room cleaned up the bite and sent George home with a prescription for an antibiotic because of the risk of infection.

But at home George had no car, no driver's license, no way to get to the pharmacy for the antibiotic.

So a week later, he was in Steph Diehlmann's clinic with an infected wound.

Between sobs, George poured out his life story. His drinking began when he was eleven years old and a child soldier against his will in the Second Sudanese Civil War. Alcohol was the only way to escape what he was forced to do, to close his eyes against what he could not unsee.

He carried the memories with him to a new country, however. When George was fourteen, he came to the United States and lived with a foster family, but still he found ways to drink and numb the horrors of having been a child soldier. Eventually he moved out, married, and had a family, and still his past and his addiction gripped him. How does anyone, especially a child, get over those kinds of mental wounds?

Now he'd lost his job, his family, his car, his driver's license, all to the unhealed trauma of a childhood most of us can't begin to imagine. That's why he couldn't do something as simple as get himself to the pharmacy and fill a prescription.

"We can help you," Steph said. "You can go to rehab. We will work on getting you some help." Steph talked with George about addiction treatments and post-traumatic stress disorder.

Then she offered to pray for him, and George nodded.

"God, may you touch George's life and take this terrible pain from him."

George's "brother," the friend who had bitten him while drunk but who was there with him, asked, "Can I pray for him too?"

"Sure!" Steph widened the circle, and the friend prayed as well.

"No Way, Lord"

Steph Diehlmann is a medical missionary, one of hundreds of medical professionals who believe there is a link between faith and health and are living out a calling to a health-care ministry. The Well, the clinic she opened in Cactus, Texas, is part of a growing network of medical facilities in the United States operating with the help of faith communities seeking to be faithful to the belief that God created us to care for both our bodies and our spirits. They provide quality health care for people in the margins of the US health-care system.

I know Steph because in 1987, as a United Methodist minister and family medicine physician, I opened Church Health in Memphis, Tennessee, to serve the working uninsured in one of the poorest cities in the country. We've grown into the largest charitably funded faith-based clinic in the country, and other people opening clinics sometimes visit our work to pick our brains. Steph had heard about us.

How did Steph become George's doctor? Why do people like Steph dedicate their careers to this type of ministry?

As a teenager, Steph went with her father on a mission trip to Nicaragua. The main purpose was to build a new library, but a couple of nurses were on the trip, and they set up a small clinic in the sanctuary of a church and asked Steph to help. With an infectious smile and perky disposition, she was eager to assist. "Give people the pills when they come to you." That was her charge. Pretty easy. But then a young mother stood in front of her with her child suffering intensely from diarrhea. The mother, not much older than Steph, held her listless infant. Steph felt helpless. She couldn't get the child's sunken face out of her mind.

On the flight home to Ohio, Steph was certain God spoke to her: "Steph, you are going to be a doctor." She was also sure God had the wrong person. "No way, Lord. I'm not going to school all those years." Or so she thought.

The voice of God never left her. She kept feeling the pull to medicine. During college—with a premed major—Steph had several more medical mission experiences, including working in a hospital in India and doing rural public health education. She was drawn to the plight of women giving birth, especially what she calls "some crazy OB stuff."

Steph went on to medical school at Ohio State and did her residency in family medicine with a strong international health focus in Fort Worth, Texas. Taking care of incoming refugees for resettlement, she learned to coach women through labor in Spanish. "¡Puje!" she would yell. "¡Puje! ¡Puje!" Push. Push. When the pushing was finished, she was there to welcome the baby. Then she went into a one-year fellowship in high-risk obstetrics. Steph knew she was on the right path, the path God had called her to take.

When her training was finished, her next move was soon clear. The Church of the Nazarene, her denomination, asked her to become a missionary in Papua New Guinea (PNG) serving as a women's health specialist. She packed up to fly halfway around the world to join seven other mission doctors in Kudjip, in the hill country of PNG.

It was a romantic setting for a two-week vacation, but it was not for the faint of heart, especially if you are a young single woman. As many as 70 percent of young women in PNG are raped at some point. It wasn't safe for Steph to walk alone. Wherever she went, she needed an escort.

Medically, her practice was both challenging and rewarding. Every conceivable obstetrical problem turned up at her clinic. Few days went by without a crisis. It was exhausting. The death of a mother or a baby was always a breath away. Low-birth-weight babies were the norm. Babies weighing less than two pounds were very common. In the United States such babies can be supported and live normal lives, but in PNG so much can go wrong. Steph devoted herself to giving both the mother and the child a chance to live.

She worked nonstop, so there was little time to consider dating—not that dating existed in any sense resembling what we understand it to be as a way to choose and grow a romantic relationship. If an unmarried woman was seen with a young man, onlookers assumed sex was involved. It was a conundrum for a missionary.

After several years in the field, Steph went home to the States to rest, speak to churches, and raise money for her work. While there, she met Andy, a plumber and pipe fitter. Andy was adventurous and attractive. He had a big personality, dark-brown hair, and blue eyes. And he was drawn to "Dokta" Steph, as she was known.

Andy had been on a mission trip to Haiti after the catastrophic earthquake in 2010. Why not check out PNG? he thought. After all, Steph was there. As it turned out, the mission had plans to build a dam nearby. It made sense for a plumber and pipe fitter to lend his skills.

It all went great, except for the no-dating rule. Any time Steph and Andy were together, they had a chaperone. No exceptions. Steph just laughed it off.

Then, like a fairytale where she was the princess, Steph and Andy went on an adventure. It ended in feathers and face paint and roasting a pig in a *mumu*, an in-ground oven. Andy asked Steph to marry her, and she said yes.

It was time to go home. Steph and Andy returned to Ohio. Steph worked in an inner-city clinic in Columbus, where for three years they waited for

God to lead them to the next place in life. That's when Cactus, Texas, came into view. In 2011, the Church of the Nazarene built a ministry center with an array of services in a small town in rural Texas.

Cactus has a population of 3,500 people. It is a center for agriculture and cattle processing, with feed lots, dairies, and a large meatpacking facility that processes five thousand head of cattle a day. It is grueling, dirty work. The workers are almost all refugees, representing twenty-six nationalities and speaking forty languages. People have come from all over the world to work in this near-desert community. The need for food programs, social services, and after-school tutoring was evident, and the church's ministry center stepped in. What was absent and sorely needed, though, was a medical clinic.

Enter Steph.

Even in jobs that offer health insurance, many refugee employees don't understand how it works. And since they are saving as much money as they can to send to family back home, even the small amount of money required for the employee's portion of health insurance seems too much, so they don't enroll. It isn't a problem until it is.

It was clear to the ministry-center staff that a medical clinic was essential, but it was also clear that it would not be as easy to start as a food pantry or clothes closet. This was far more complicated and required expertise they didn't have.

Steph and Andy knew they were being called to Cactus to continue to live out a medical mission linking faith and health. Steph could do the doctoring, obviously. With Andy's expertise they could fix facility problems as they arose. What they didn't know how to do was run a clinic administratively. Hiring people, training people, firing people if necessary. Raising money. Setting up human resources regulations. Purchasing. The list went on and on. Starting a clinic and being an administrator wasn't anything Steph had ever trained to do.

Nevertheless, they moved to Cactus in late 2017 with a passion. Now what?

Looking God in the Face

In the process of uncovering resources, Steph heard about Church Health, the primary care clinic I began from scratch in 1987, and Empowering

Church Health Outreach (ECHO), an organization that helps create new full-service health clinics based on our model. Steph began to see how things could all come together. She sponged up knowledge and couldn't learn fast enough. There was no question that with her passion, the clinic she would call The Well would work. With the backing of the Church of the Nazarene, Steph went to Cactus and began the heavy lifting. Nothing like this is ever easy. She got a $20,000 start-up grant. She found a way to get laboratory tests done at reasonable rates. She tackled all the obstacles one by one. About two hundred volunteers, divided into twenty teams, built a clinic inside a multipurpose room, and they opened in January of 2019.

The patients started to come, and they continue to come.

Steph was able to arrange transportation for George to get the anti-biotic he needed. George returned a week after Steph first saw him, and his infected finger looked a lot better. Steph tried to address his PTSD again, but George wasn't ready to talk about seeing a counselor to help him stop drinking. She scheduled another appointment, thinking maybe more time might bring him around, but he never returned. Steph could only assume he was still struggling with the horrors of his past, his addiction, and all the compounded losses in his life.

But Steph is not discouraged. She named the clinic The Well because Jesus is the Living Water and is a supply that never dries up, not even in a place like Cactus.

Steph thinks of Cactus as similar to Samaria, where Jesus encountered the woman at the well. Samaria was considered what Steph calls a rubbish kind of place full of outcasts. "That is what people think of Cactus," she says. "Of course this is where we should be ministering in Jesus's name."

Steph prays that George will come back to see her and take the next step in healing more than his finger. Until then, remembering that the Lord is close to the brokenhearted and saves those who are crushed in spirit, she says, "We will pray he will come back to us. And we will keep doing the work."

While Steph and I are about three decades apart in our experiences of launching faith-based health-care clinics that serve vulnerable popu-lations, we have both confronted the fundamental truth that our work is complex. The US health-care system can be daunting enough for those of us who have good jobs, steady incomes, and health insurance. What hap-pens when one of those stakes is absent? Or two? Or all three? Health and health care begin to take on an entirely different shape, one that looks less like a well-constructed house and more like a tent tied up at the corners because the poles went missing. George's story hit me in the gut because he could be one of my own patients—or several rolled together. An immigrant. A past riddled with trauma that follows him wherever he goes. No insurance. Unstable employment. No regular doctor. No transportation to get something as simple as an antibiotic. Addiction issues. Not ready or able to catch the lifeline thrown to him in love.

If George doesn't challenge us to wrestle with what it means for people of faith to put legs on the healing message of the gospel Jesus taught, what will? If you are not a doctor, you might ask, "What can I do to make a difference in the health of people who fall through the cracks?" Starting a clinic might be impossible. Still, the call to discipleship and following Jesus is clear: preach, teach—and heal.

Do any of us, at the end of time, really want to look God in the face and have God say, "Did you think I was kidding about that?"

What Jesus Shows Us about Health

John Wesley shocked the living daylights out of people.

Not literally. But public demonstrations of electricity were popular in the mid-eighteenth century. Portable machines astonished crowds by using friction electricity to ignite ether or brandy with sparks from people's fingers. John Wesley was infatuated.

Wesley's fascination with shocking people started with Benjamin Franklin, who could have killed himself flying a kite with an iron key attached to it during a thunderstorm. But he lived to write pamphlets about electricity, and John Wesley studied them. From there it was a short leap to wondering how electricity might be useful in healing physical conditions. Wesley got himself a machine and first shocked himself to treat his own ailing leg. Seeing some gradual improvement in his condition, he began offering electric shock to others through the free clinics he operated. Thousands of people tried electric shock. Wesley kept meticulous records and eventually identified thirty-seven disorders he believed responded to the treatment. And in cases where the treatment did not help, he didn't believe it caused any harm.

Wesley is most famous as a minister and the founder of Methodism, the origin of the Methodist Church. What is less well-known is that Wesley practiced medicine from the age of nineteen until he died. This was part and parcel of his ministry and his view of the world, particularly demonstrated in the health care he offered to the poor. Wesley typically traveled about fifty thousand miles a year around the English countryside on horseback, and he was as interested in healing physical ailments as he was in preaching and promoting Methodist societies. In taking this stance, Wesley joined a long Christian tradition of caring for both body and spirit.

The enfleshing of Jesus, God's own Son, says something of what God thinks of being human. God created the physical world and called it "good." God created human beings and said, "*Very* good." Then God gave Jesus human birth, human flesh, human experience.

Jesus slept when he was tired, walked everywhere he went, sat on hillsides, anticipated questions, told stories, paid taxes, stroked the heads of children, loved his own mother, made his siblings wait, experienced temptation, cried over the death of a close friend, acted with compassion, enjoyed good meals, debated with cultural leaders, talked to people he "should have known better" than to be seen with, pointed out the errors of his best friends, washed dirty feet.

Jesus lived life within the confines and disappointments of a body. John writes in a more theological style than the other three gospel writers of the New Testament, but even his starting point is that Jesus took on flesh. The Word of God—God's own Son—became human and lived a human life among other humans. While he lived on earth, Jesus was not just a spiritual being hiding in a physical body. He was flesh and blood. He was human. God created humanity, including the body, and did not hesitate to send Jesus to experience what we experience. That tells us something about what God thinks of the human body.

Jesus lived a life of faith connected to God. He never drifted away from this anchor. Being human and living in a human body did not separate Jesus from God. Being human put Jesus right where God wanted him to be, to do the work God wanted him to do. Jesus's ministry included preaching to the crowds, teaching his followers, and healing people whose bodies failed them—in order to show God's power at work. He healed people whose legs were lame, whose ears were deaf, whose eyes were blind, whose skin was leprous, whose spirits were demon possessed. He even healed dead people. Jesus cared about bodies because he cared about the whole person in relationship to God. Living a life of faith in the body is not just for Jesus. God wants this for all of us.

The Gospel Call to Heal

I first came to Memphis in 1986. Having completed my theological and medical education, I was determined to begin a health-care ministry for the working uninsured in low-wage jobs. I had dreamed of this for years as I slogged my way through the training that would make it possible. When the time came, I chose Memphis because historically it is one of the poorest major cities in the United States. Today we see patients in clinics for primary care, urgent care, dental work, and optometry services. Behavioral health, life coaching, and physical rehabilitation are integrated into our clinics, and we have a teaching kitchen offering classes on culinary medicine for patients and the community.

God calls the church to healing work. Jesus's life was about healing the whole person, and Jesus is the church in the world. Jesus's message is our message. Jesus's ministry is our ministry. As a community, then, how do we look at the eyes of our neighbors, listen to their stories, and together seek the solutions that invite everyone into God's wellness?

The early church went from scattered disciples after Jesus's resurrection to being the official religion of the Roman Empire in the fourth century. That didn't happen only because of great preaching. During the second and third centuries, as plagues spread across the Roman world, it was the Christians who were willing to care for the sick. When people recovered, Romans asked, "Who is your God that I might worship him?"

This is the God who called a girl in Ohio to be a medical missionary.

George in Cactus, Texas, challenges me.

And Steph, following God's voice from Ohio to PNG to Cactus, inspires me.

Emergencies like the COVID-19 pandemic challenge me with all the inequality it exposed in readiness, access to care, and outcomes among particular groups of vulnerable people.

That's what this book is about—people who challenge us to see what Jesus saw when he reached out to heal and people who inspire us to believe that in answering Jesus's call together, what we do matters for our own discipleship and for the lives of people God puts in our paths.

We start with understanding the context of the lives of people who work hard and don't have health insurance or access to health care they can afford. You'll read a lot of stories in this book. That's the best way I know to help you meet the people Stephanie Diehlmann and I—and others—meet every day and step into their lives for a few minutes. And then let's figure out how to do the work of Jesus together.

For Reflection

1. What was your earliest experience of having a sense of what God's call might be for your life?
2. Have you ever met anyone with a complex past like George with so many needs? What was the impact on you?
3. How does a community like Cactus, Texas, compare to where you live? In what ways might the people in Cactus and in your community be more alike than different?

TWO

FLIPPING BETWEEN A LIVING AND HEALTH CARE

Rarecas Williams came in the back door carrying a box he was delivering to me for Jack Phillips. He was a muscular thirty-year-old who was not very tall, but as soon as he entered, he fell while holding the box. He didn't trip; he just collapsed. He struggled to get back up. It was clear something wasn't right.

"You need to come see me," I told him, not knowing who he was other than that he was helping Jack.

"I'm fine," he said. Then after he took a couple of more steps, he fell again.

"No, I'm serious. You need to come see me."

"Yes, sir, I will."

I told Jack his friend had a problem we needed to figure out. He told me he would make sure Rarecas saw me.

In a couple of days, he appeared on the schedule. I walked in unsure what trouble I would find. Rarecas immediately spoke up with what I would come to recognize as his bigger-than-life personality.

"My problem is I got shot in the butt."

That was an interesting opening line. "When did that happen?" I asked.

"About a year ago. The bullet's still in there." He showed me where the bullet was lodged.

I asked him to get undressed so I could examine him. He struggled to do so and get on the exam table. This was something more than a bullet wound to his backside. His arms were weak, and he had developed muscle wasting in his legs. When I checked the reflexes in his legs, he almost kicked me after I barely touched his knee. This was not good.

"Doc, I am having trouble flipping," he said.

I didn't know what he meant, but soon I figured out who Rarecas is, and I felt privileged to be taking care of him. He is the original Beale Street Flipper.

In 1986, when he was five years old, Rarecas, or Rod, lived with his mother and her nine other children, plus his father and five more of his father's children in a three-bedroom house at the end of Pontotoc Street near downtown Memphis.

After the Civil War, Beale Street began attracting a variety of Black entrepreneurs along with blues musicians. Robert Church became the city's first Black millionaire and was based on Beale Street. At the turn of the century, W. C. Handy became famous playing on the street and spawned a number of other talented musicians. Growing up on Beale Street, B. B. King became known as the Beale Street "Blues Boy"—"B. B."

In the 1960s the street fell on hard times and was known only for crime and drugs. In the 1970s the City of Memphis decided to redevelop the street as an entertainment district. By the mid-1980s, clubs had reopened and Beale Street was again seeing life. However, at the east end of the street and just one block off of it, not everyone was benefiting from the influx of capital. One block from where Rod lived was a spot the *Wall Street Journal* declared to be the "intersection of poverty and despair." In 1986, at the age of five, Rod and his friends walked over to Beale Street and Fourth Avenue. Thirty kids and forty adults gathered while a band played. Someone who had seen him do it before told Rod, "Do a flip for me," which Rod was quick to do. A White man Rod had never seen before was so impressed he came up and put a gold ring on his finger. Seeing the excitement, Rod's family set out two large empty "chitlin buckets," the type grocery stores sold. Chitlins, or chitterlings, are a prepared food made from the small intestine of a pig and are a very common inexpensive meal in the South and in Black culture. The buckets were quickly filled as Rod continued to flip.

On that day the Beale Street Flipper was born.

The next day, Rod saw his mother counting the change from the buckets. He asked her, "Mom, can I have fifty cents to go to the candy lady?"

"Son," she said enthusiastically, "you can have whatever you want."

With fifteen children in the house, Rod's mother had never given him anything, so from that day on, he went to Beale Street every day with an empty chitlin bucket. Up until 1991, it wasn't legal to flip on Beale Street, so whenever he went, there was always a four-person crew: one to guard the bucket, one to watch out for the police, and two to flip.

When he was eleven, Rod was outside of B. B. King's restaurant when a man approached him and said someone was waiting for him at the Rum Boogie Café. Rod reluctantly walked over. Sitting at the bar was a White man smoking a cigar. Rod recalled, "He never looked at me once, but he said, 'There are movie people looking for a flipper. Go over to the third floor of the Radisson Hotel. They are waiting on you. Do you understand me, son?'"

Rod had no idea what this was all about, but when he got to the Radisson, the cameras were everywhere, and they were focused on him. He was cast in the movie *The Firm*, based on John Grisham's novel.

He remembers filming the movie. "We didn't have a phone, so every day Tom Cruise sent a limo to get me." Rod's role in *The Firm* made him a Memphis icon.

Afterward he kept flipping on Beale Street and was often hired for special events, especially basketball games. As he got older, he began training other kids to flip. He chose kids who were athletic but small like he was. His goal was to keep them out of gangs and away from the drug trade rampant in his neighborhood by giving them enough money that they wouldn't be lured into being a lookout for older teens selling drugs.

On September 3, 2004, he was a few blocks off Beale when he walked past a couple of older men. One of them went by the nickname "38," after the type of gun he always carried. As Rod walked by, 38 yelled at him, "Any niggers who come around here playing are going to get shot." Rod jokingly said to him, "I have twenty kids," referring to the number of flippers working for him at the time. The next thing he knew one of the men held him by the face and turned his head. And without warning, Rod was shot.

Rod was treated at the "Med," the regional public hospital, and released, but several bullet fragments remained lodged in him. Today's manufactured bullets are often designed to break into many pieces when they penetrate the body. It seems counterintuitive that a doctor would leave the bullet in, but more often than not, the surgeon will do more harm than good by going in to get a bullet fragment than by just leaving it where it is if it is not in a dangerous place. The adage "Let sleeping dogs lie" applies here.

In most cases, the bullet will not cause any harm as long as it doesn't move. In some cases, though, it will start to migrate toward areas that give limited resistance. A bullet may even head toward the surface and can be felt by rubbing the skin. The fragments can also move toward nerves and begin to cause more damage. Rod had a hard time, as most of us would, becoming comfortable with knowing there were bullet fragments sitting in his body, even though they were not causing further damage. Multiple bullet fragments may have caused irritation, but this was not the reason for his pain.

For Rod, the primary source of his pain and nerve damage came from the fractures in his spine brought on by flipping. He never sought help because he knew he was uninsured and didn't believe anyone would be willing to help him. He still saw himself as one of fifteen children vying for his mother's favor. With little appreciation for how serious and complicated his problem was, he was just hoping and praying it would all be okay one day. His is a common prayer for people who are not used to turning to doctors for help and feel that when they do, their problems are not a priority for doctors who know their financial options are limited. All too often, the message they receive is that they need to move on because they can't afford the care offered to people with good insurance.

Rod remembers the first time I treated him after he fell in our clinic. He said, "I kept telling you that I had gotten shot in the butt, and you said to me, 'Let's not talk about your butt. That's not what the problem is.' I guess you were right."

After examining him in the clinic, I knew he had a significant problem with his spine. I immediately ordered an MRI. What it showed was like nothing I have ever seen. Every last vertebra in his back was damaged. Along with damage to the bones, the more troubling issue was with his spinal cord itself. The radiologist read it as "thoracic cord atrophy." The spinal cord was beyond repair.

I called one of our volunteer neurosurgeons, Dr. Jeff Sorensen, who immediately agreed to see Rod. Dr. Sorensen did surgery to stabilize Rod's spine, but he would never flip again. The real question was whether he would ever walk again.

Over the next few years, Rod struggled with the reality that flipping had almost certainly caused the extensive damage to his spine and spinal cord. He continued to manage the Beale Street Flippers, and I wondered if these other young people were at risk for the same thing happening to them. On several occasions I worried whether I should be examining the kids Rod was recruiting to be flippers. Was it inevitable that flipping down a city street would affect all of them? Was it just that Rod was extreme in the way he flipped and ignored injuries when they occurred? Was his body just prone to the injuries he had? I told Rod I had concerns about the kids.

He shrugged it off. "Oh, Doc. Don't worry. They're all fine. This is just me."

"But Rod," I said, "do you think the same thing might happen to them that has happened to you?"

He laughed. "Doc, you don't know what it's like to grow up where I'm from. They'll be fine."

No matter what, I was not going to get the chance to examine the other flippers. They had to make money somehow. At least they were not in gangs.

Then one day, I was seeing Rod, and he wasn't his usual upbeat self. "What's going on?"

"One of my boys got shot last night."

"What!" I was startled. "What happened?"

"Somebody lured him behind one of the clubs and tried to rob him. When he wouldn't give them anything, they shot him."

I stupidly asked, "Is he okay?"

Rod shook his head. "Nah, Doc, he's not okay."

That night my wife, Mary, and I were driving to an event downtown. We passed by a church close to where Rod grew up. A large crowd was coming and going from the church. I later realized that this was the visitation for Rod's flipper who had been killed. Rod knew far better than I that the risks of flipping were more serious than just an injury to the back. But the risks to not earning an income were higher.

Rod's problems got worse. He crossed his legs one day while lying in bed and he heard a crack. This time the MRI notes for his right hip said, "Complete destruction of the femoral head." The bone that forms the main part of what we call the hip had been irreparably broken. There was no way it would heal on its own. His hip would never work correctly again. What more could go wrong?

Rod became depressed. He and his wife separated. He started buying drugs on the street to deal with the pain.

Thankfully our mutual friend Jack kept hiring him to work at one of his restaurants and stayed with him for support.

In the middle of his worst times, Rod called to make an appointment with me, only in doing so he cursed out our phone operator and threatened to come down and hurt her. He crossed the line.

"Rod, what you did was unacceptable. You can't come here anymore," I told him.

He didn't argue. "I know I shouldn't have done that. I was wrong."

I felt he was sincere, but I still had to protect our staff.

Time went on and I wondered how he was doing. Jack called and asked, "Can you call in the medicine that helps with his spasticity? I understand if you can't."

I paused. "He can come to the walk-in clinic and I will see him. But he has to be on his best behavior."

And so I am back to seeing Rod. He is confined to a wheelchair. He can't move his right leg at all. He still has a big laugh. His wife has moved back in with him.

"I took a look at myself and I didn't like what I saw," he said. "It is all about respect."

It took me a minute to understand what he meant, but it seemed that he had come to realize that the relationship with his wife couldn't just be about her taking care of him. It takes two to make a relationship. He is finally coming to see how a marriage works. But his comment about respect also seemed to be addressed to me.

No one in Memphis knows what happened to the Beale Street Flipper. They see his kids flip anytime they go down Beale Street. They still put money in the chitlin buckets, and he is off to the side in his wheelchair with his big smile, but where is the respect for him?

Sometimes my staff, I think, believe that I have cut Rod too much slack. He has at times been overly demanding to the people on the phone or at the front desk, and I keep giving him another chance. I see their point. I think part of my leniency is assuaging my own sense of guilt.

For many years I was like so many others whenever I saw the Beale Street Flippers. I loved their show. If I was with people from out of town and we were walking down Beale Street and I saw the flippers performing, I would go out of my way to take guests over to see the show. I realized the flippers worked for tips, but I know that on more occasions than not I walked by the chitlin bucket without putting anything in. I took pride in knowing that Rod and his boys created a unique act for Memphis but too often failed to think about him or his boys as people. I, like I suspect most, loved the show but didn't consider the person. The flippers were amazing, but did they ever fall? What happened if they did? Surely no one would try to steal the chitlin bucket. I just didn't think beyond the moments of entertainment to what happened to the performers.

Of course the question is, Should I have been more concerned? I was just walking down Beale Street and there they were. They were making money from their tips. As far as I know, they made far more than they would have working minimum wage, and maybe more importantly, more than working for drug lords.

But it is not just the flippers. We have chance encounters with so many people who are doing things that entertain us or make our lives easier but whose health issues don't concern us. If Jesus calls us to healing ministry as a way to follow him, shouldn't we be willing to at least embrace the notion that the flippers' health care is something that the church and faith community should be aware of, if not actively trying to engage?

Turning Heads

Just before walking into the exam room, I told Brian, who was shadowing me, "See this paper? It's from a lawyer trying to get this patient on disability. I don't fill out papers for lawyers. All they want is the money if the patient is approved."

Brian and I then entered the room. When I saw Lillian, my mouth almost dropped open. I had never seen anything quite like what I was looking at. A Black woman in her early fifties with short black hair and dressed professionally, she began talking to me in an upbeat fashion—although her head was turned as far to the left as it was possible to turn. Then she asked me, "Do you think you can move over a little so I can see you?"

Sheepish, I said, "Of course," and walked three steps to my right. She smiled at me and we continued to talk.

She would later say to me, "If it wasn't for my shoulder, I think my head would just keep on turning." Lillian had a condition I have almost never seen, known as torticollis. For no good reason, the muscles on the left side of her neck contract continuously and will not release and allow her to move her head in any way. She continually looks to her left, and the constant tension is quite painful.

I looked at the papers in my hand from the lawyer, embarrassed at what I had said to Brian, and began asking her questions as though I saw her problem every day. It had begun slowly at first almost five years earlier, but two years ago it had gotten severe. Looking at our records, I saw she had come to our walk-in clinic about that time. One of our other providers had seen her and ordered physical therapy. She had never gone. I asked why.

She matter-of-factly replied, "Because I was told I didn't qualify to be a patient here. I wasn't working."

My stomach sank. That was technically right—our mission is to serve the *working* uninsured. Anyone can come to our walk-in clinic for urgent care, as Lillian initially had, but becoming a regular patient requires working twenty hours a week or more. But I have always said that we have guidelines, not rules, and we do make exceptions. We don't always get it right.

In the years since we'd seen her, Lillian had tried to see several doctors, none of whom knew what to do for her. Just the previous week, after a long wait, she had seen a neurologist through the university.

I was upbeat to hear that. "What did she tell you?"

"She told me my case was more than she knew what to do with. She referred me to the dystonia clinic at Vanderbilt. But I can't be seen there because I am uninsured."

It was a vicious circle of evident medical need and a lack of resources and mismatched qualifying criteria.

Lillian was with a friend who clearly cared for her deeply, a slightly older woman in her sixties.

She jumped in. "I will pay for the visit if we can just get her seen."

I could feel desperation.

I then leaned over to both of them and said, "We will find the best doctor in Memphis to take care of you, and if we have to go to Vanderbilt in Nashville, we will plead your case." I could feel them sigh.

Then I realized that Dr. Victoria Lim was literally just outside the door working as a volunteer head-and-neck surgeon for us that morning. The person I needed might be ten feet away.

I told Lillian to stay put while I went and got Victoria. She came in and began an examination. I knew that Lillian's problem was something that Victoria had also rarely seen.

When we both stepped outside to confer, Victoria said she didn't think that she was the right person to treat Lillian, but she had a couple of ideas of people in Memphis who could help. We both thought a trial of injecting Botox in her neck was worth the effort.

These days, Botox is most well-known for its cosmetic use in temporarily relieving facial wrinkles. I suspect people wouldn't so freely inject it into their faces if they knew what it is. But it is also used therapeutically for a number of conditions.

Botox is shorthand for botulinum toxin type A and is a toxin extracted from the bacteria that causes botulism, which can be life-threatening. In cosmetic use, Botox paralyzes muscles so they are unable to contract. Wrinkles smooth out because the toxin effectively poisons the nerve. A very small dose is injected, so after a few months the nerve can be revived, but if too much were to be injected, the paralysis could be permanent. It's used for treating chronic migraine and other disorders. The drug was created at first for the purpose of treating problems like Lillian's. She was in fact the perfect candidate for Botox.

When I asked Lillian if she would be up to trying it, she didn't hesitate. "I will try anything. This is no way to live."

Botox for therapeutic uses is not cheap, though. It can run into hundreds or thousands of dollars for a single treatment.

Lillian's friend quickly said, "I'll pay for it."

Dr. Lim and I decided on the specialist we wanted Lillian to see. He had been a volunteer for Church Health in the past, and I was confident I could get him to see her. I was less confident that he could solve the problem, but at least we had a start. In the meantime, Dr. Lim and I agreed that we should see if a course of strong steroids could offer any relief.

I told Lillian, "I think you should take prednisone for now until you see the specialist. Are you okay with that?"

Without blinking she replied, "I don't know. Won't those things make me fat?"

I could feel myself tensing up over her worrying about that.

Then she smiled. "I got you, Doc. I'm just kidding. Of course I want to try it if you think it could help."

She had indeed gotten me, but in doing so she fully won me over to her cause.

While the first order of business was to find a treatment, it was also important to get Lillian on disability. That, after all, was the main reason she had come. She had applied for disability twice and been turned down.

"They told me that my hands and feet work, so I should be able to work."

I was not surprised. She had not had a physician advocate for her, and even if she had, she might have been turned down. The system is truly dysfunctional.

The lawyers she had contacted would help her appeal her case, and if they succeeded, they would take the first couple of payments as their fee. It takes little effort on their part to file the paperwork. I emphatically answered the questions on the disability form in the affirmative, stating that she was unable to work.

What I knew would come next was the lawyers' wanting me to do more, none of which would Church Health be paid for, even though the lawyers would be compensated. But for once, I didn't care. I would eagerly fill out more forms and even testify on Lillian's behalf if needed. This was because I felt guilty that we turned her away two years earlier. Thankfully, her friend gave me dispensation.

As I apologized for our not helping her two years ago, Lillian said, "We will only look forward. We are grateful for your help today."

It would be a long road, but I was now committed to walking it with her.

Dueling Genealogies

"Asa Candler approached my great-grandfather in 1892 and asked him to become a partner in manufacturing a new elixir."

With some pride, I shared this tidbit of family history with Billy Warren, a new friend I was just getting to know. I was in the eighth grade and had just started as a student at the Westminster Schools in Atlanta, an affluent private school in Buckhead, the wealthiest neighborhood in the city.

Asa Candler was a druggist who became intrigued with an elixir made partly from the coca leaves from which cocaine is extracted. Candler's plan was to market the drink as a treatment for mental and physical fatigue and as a cure for headaches. With the cocaine content, I can see why people might think it could do all that and more.

When Billy and I had this conversation, the school year had not quite started. We were both on the eighth-grade football team, and practice began two weeks before the first class. Billy had been at Westminster since the first grade, but I was a newbie. I was excited to be the team's quarterback, and I could tell we would be competitive, mostly because of the new kids on the squad. It was hard on people like Billy—it seemed to me—because he might not play as much as he was used to. I wasn't accustomed to such affluence and was awkwardly trying to fit in by throwing around a name like Asa Candler.

Westminster opened in 1951, before the Supreme Court's decision in *Brown v. Board of Education* in 1954 and in the era when Atlanta was severely segregated. The court's decision would not have applied to private schools, and it was more than a decade after *Brown v. Board of Education* that Westminster voluntarily considered the question of a few Black students. My class, starting in the eighth grade, was to be the first integrated class. One of the first Black students was Jannard Wade, who played end on the football team. He was tall and had good hands. Since I was the quarterback, he would be the main person I would throw to, so of course we needed to become friends, and we did.

Billy and I were also starting to become friends in the locker room and after practice. He was not very big physically, but he was tough and played hard. He had thick blond hair and a big smile. He also liked to talk. The story about Asa Candler came from my grandfather, who was a true entrepreneur. He also had a tendency to tell a story the way he wanted to, whether it fit the truth or not. The end of the story is that my great-grandfather refused to invest in Asa Candler's elixir. Of course the drink turned out to be Coca-Cola.

Billy listened intently to my tale with a wry smile and took in everything I was saying. When I was finished, he said, "That's quite a story."

I thought it was. That's why I told it.

Then Billy said, "My great-great-grandfather *was* Asa Candler."

Whoosh. The air went out of that balloon. Despite my embarrassment over trying to impress someone whose family had created and grown the

Coca-Cola empire, Billy and I became friends. Billy's slight build eventually meant that he didn't play football all the way through school, but he cheered from the sidelines when we won the state championship during our senior year. The person who turned out to be the best player was Jannard. I was proud of my friend.

When we graduated, our baccalaureate speaker was Dr. William Holmes Borders, a Black pastor and activist in the civil rights movement in Atlanta. At the time, the significance of this choice was lost on me, but I came to see it made sense for him to mark the day of Jannard's graduation. While I don't remember the content of his sermon, I do remember one moment. After preaching for about twenty minutes, he stopped mid-sentence and said, "I see all of you White folks out there looking at your watches and thinking since it is almost noon I must be about finished, but what you have never understood is that the Holy Spirit never arrives until twelve thirty." After that he continued preaching, barely taking a breath for the next forty-five minutes.

After graduation I lost touch with both Jannard and Billy. We went to different colleges, and we each moved down our own paths.

Or so I thought.

When I was a third-year medical student at Emory School of Medicine, I spent most of my rotations at Grady Hospital in downtown Atlanta. As an institution, Grady was very old. It first opened in 1892 with a hundred beds divided equally between serving Blacks and Whites. Just before World War I, the hospital expanded and separated into two facilities, Blacks in one and Whites in another. This was when this hospital first became known as the "Gradys"—plural. In the 1940s, plans began to build a sixteen-story, thousand-bed hospital with architecture in the shape of an *H* that carefully supported segregation. The front wings would serve White patients and face the city, while the back wings would serve Black patients and clearly be a back entrance. Only one hallway of the *H* connected the long wings. World War II delayed construction, and by the time the war was over and the economy and construction had revved up again, many advised abandoning the segregated architecture because they believed institutional segregation could not last much longer even in the South. But the superintendent at the time was adamantly committed to it, promising that the hospital would not be integrated in his lifetime. Construction began in 1954, and the new hospital—still called the "Gradys" because of the continued separation—opened in 1958. The facilities were designed mostly equal but definitely separate. There were two of everything. Two operating rooms, two emergency rooms, two wards, and so on. Even the laundry was done on different days so the sheets would not be mixed up, and the nursing staff was separate.

In 1965, integration was required for institutions to receive federal funds. Since the superintendent who had held out for so many years had died the year before, the hospital quickly complied. By 1982, when I was a student there, Grady was simply the hospital for the poor, Black or White. But the architecture of segregation remained. It was complicated for physicians to walk from one floor to the other. Stairwells only opened on every other floor so that you did not easily end up where you did not belong in the days of segregation. Sometimes we had to go up or down past the floor we were trying to get to and go a long way out of our paths across the *H* to see our patients. The two ERs, previously divided along racial lines, were reassigned as a surgical ER and a medical ER. The staff referred to both as the "Saturday Night Knife and Gun Club." Patients were meant to be learning tools, and it never felt to me like their humanity was the first priority.

While on my pediatric rotation, I was in the staff cafeteria one day when I looked across the room and saw Billy Warren. Pleasantly surprised, I walked over and said, "My lord, what are you doing here?"

"I'm a doctor," he responded. "What are you doing here?"

Since I had gone to seminary after college before enrolling in medical school, Billy was three years ahead of me in his medical training, so he was a second-year pediatric resident. This meant that for the next month he would be my boss.

It was a busy month, and we had little time to catch up, but he was interested in my being a Methodist minister and my plans for a church-based health clinic. He had become a devoted Christian with decidedly evangelical theology since I had known him. Billy never lacked in confidence, so when we discussed issues where I thought there was a lot of gray, Billy was far more assured. After a while it seemed best not to talk very much about Jesus.

As I was finishing medical school and heading to Virginia for my family medicine residency, Billy told me that he had decided to practice pediatrics in Sandy Springs, the community in Atlanta where I grew up. By then Sandy Springs had become known as the "Golden Ghetto." Billy was going to be a suburban pediatrician. Since I was planning to open a clinic to serve the poor, I figured we probably would not be seeing much of each other except at Westminster reunions.

And then in 1995, more than a decade later, Billy changed his course. He began a part-time pediatric clinic in a distressed part of Atlanta and named it Good Samaritan. At first he just worked out of one room in a church. Then in 1998 he took the plunge. He left his successful practice in Sandy Springs to open Good Samaritan Health Center in a very poor neighborhood near Georgia Tech. By then I had been in Memphis leading Church Health for over a decade, and he came to visit us and see our work. I was impressed with the decision he made, but I was worried about one thing. How can the great-great-grandson of Asa Candler, an heir to Coca-Cola, raise money to run a clinic for the poor?

I have never been burdened with being an heir to anything, but the question reflects the challenge of doing anything that requires people sharing their wealth for the good of others. I'm sure Billy constantly runs into people expecting him to just fund the entire operation. That is impossible and certainly not sustainable. But it requires much of him to be willing to listen to such thoughts and remain thoroughly engaged with wanting to provide a full, rich service to those Good Sam serves. Billy, or Dr. Bill Warren, as everyone now knows him, can't do it alone.

In 2009 Good Sam expanded once again. It has grown beyond limiting services to pediatric care, Bill's original specialty, to offering an array of services. The medical care they provide includes primary care for the whole family, with prenatal care and specialty services through volunteer physicians. The uninsured, low-income patients who come to Good Sam also receive dental care and behavioral health services, including same-day assessments when needed, along with scheduled counseling sessions. A health-education program addresses the nutritional and lifestyle needs of individuals with diabetes and offers cooking classes. They have even begun growing fruits and vegetables that patients and guests can buy at prices they can afford in the middle of a food desert. The organization fosters community partnerships with schools, shelters, recovery organizations, and housing resources that can help meet the nonmedical needs of people living in poverty. The vast majority of their patients have no form of medical insurance. In some ways, the racial issues that stood in the way of access to care a hundred years ago at the Gradys are still a factor in Atlanta. Over 90 percent of patients at Good Sam—low income with no insurance—are non-Caucasian. Too often families face choices between basics, like food and shelter, and paying for health care.

The Beale Street Flipper certainly did. And I still worry that other kids who are flipping are endangering their long-term health because flipping is how they can make money to cover basic expenses *now*. The Good Samaritan Health Center wants to remove the burden of that choice by serving people who have the least access to care and the highest risk of serious health issues.

Good Sam is my kind of place, and I know Steph Diehlmann would say the same. Their motivation is the same as ours at Church Health and the same as The Well in Cactus, Texas—living the call of the gospel by following Jesus through health care for the uninsured and underinsured people working at low-wage jobs.

The Story in Numbers

Rod Williams grew up poor and learned, of necessity, to focus on immediate financial needs. Relative to housing, food, utilities, and transportation, insurance premiums didn't qualify. Lillian was caught in systems very good at screening people out rather than including them, despite the obvious need sitting right in front of us. Neither of them could be called lazy, and they asked for very little, actually. People who work with as much dignity as Rod and Lillian yet who always seem to be on the outside of health care fill the clinics at places like Church Health and Good Samaritan.

Prior to the Affordable Care Act (ACA), the number of uninsured in the United States had grown to forty-six million. As of 2021, even with all the people who have found plans through the ACA, that number sits at over twenty-nine million and is growing by about one million a year.[1] The primary reason people are uninsured is no surprise—cost. In 2021, the cost of premiums and deductibles for a family of four averaged $28,256 according to the Milliman Medical Index. Even subtracting the portion that an employer bears on average, this leaves $12,249 for the family to cover out of pocket for premiums, deductibles, and copays. And from 2010 to 2020, the worker's share of premiums increased by 40 percent, certainly a higher rate than wages increased during this period of time. The percent-age of income a family at the lower end of the economic spectrum spends on insurance premiums and out-of-pocket costs is obviously significantly higher than families living above the poverty level.[2] The annual income of someone making $12 an hour and working full-time is $24,960. (At Church Health, 90 percent of our patients earn less than $12 an hour.) Federal subsidies to offset the cost of premiums of policies under the ACA are not equally available in every state. In some states, people who earn less than the poverty line cannot qualify for subsidized private insurance, but nei-ther do they qualify for Medicaid. In 2019, nearly 74 percent of uninsured adults who are not yet old enough to qualify for Medicare said the cost of insurance is the reason they are uninsured.[3]

Of those who were uninsured in 2019, 84 percent were part of a house-hold where someone was working full-time. Some employees in low-wage jobs who have the option of employer-provided insurance won't always take it because even then the employee portion of the premium and high deductibles take too big a bite out of the family paycheck. But a large ma-jority of uninsured working adults, 72.5 percent, do not have access to an employer plan. As a proportion of the general population, people of color are more at risk of being uninsured than White individuals. People without insurance are less likely to receive preventive care for chronic conditions and are more likely to postpone needed care because of cost—30 percent compared to about 5 percent of adults with private coverage—or to not fill a prescription they need—nearly 20 percent compared to 6 percent. Seventy-seven percent of the uninsured are US citizens.[4] These are the faces of the uninsured in the United States and the impact lack of insurance has on their care.

About 1,400 free and charitable clinics across the United States care for 2.9 million patients with 6.9 million visits annually. They do this with the help of 207,600 volunteers and 106,500 medical providers according to the National Association for Free and Charitable Clinics. The average one-time cost of an emergency room visit, where many uninsured people end up even for non-emergencies simply because they don't have regular doctors, is $1,389. Free and charitable clinics that see uninsured patients save $9.6 bil-lion a year in ER charges for which hospitals might not be compensated or which would mire the uninsured in medical debt. Fifty-two percent of these clinics have a budget of less than $250,000 a year, yet on average every dollar they spend translates into a value of five dollars' worth of care.[5]

Running after God's Priorities

Bill Warren and I are still in different places when it comes to the details of our theology, but as we have gotten older, we both see that God's kingdom is bigger than just one approach. None of us has all the answers alone. We need each other. And the work has to go on beyond any one city or leader's life span. The type of work done by Good Sam in Atlanta, Church Health in Memphis, and The Well in Cactus, serving the underserved because our faith calls us to do so, requires the full commitment of rich and poor and of the whole church.

I might never know if the Beale Street Flipper's spine would have been susceptible to damage from other life issues if he hadn't been doing back flips on sidewalks when he was five. But I do know that his life circumstances in general would have kept health care out of his financial reach. He needed an advocate like Jack to point him to where he could get care and people of faith who were ready to provide it. And would Lillian's condition be less advanced if her being unemployed because of it had not gotten in the way of receiving care she certainly could not afford to pay for?

Across the United States there are faith-based free and charitable clinics like The Well, Good Samaritan, and Church Health. As a physician in one of these clinics, I can tell somebody like Rod to come and see me or try to make things right for someone like Lillian. In my experience, most Christians in ordinary congregations have no idea they may be worshiping a few miles away from a health clinic that takes care of Rod or Lillian or George. I do know you don't have to be a medical professional to help.

Find out what already exists in your community and get to know the people who have dedicated their lives to the mission of health care for the vulnerable. You don't have to become a health clinic administrator, and your church doesn't have to start a clinic—unless that's your specific calling—but you can put your arms around a local clinic and support it as your own. Yes, clinics need financial support, but they also need so much else. Discover what. Recruit volunteers for the clinic. Organize work teams to rehab expanded space. Coordinate with other congregations. Match expertise to the needs.

The book of Acts in the New Testament is full of miraculous healings, and the early church also expected healing would come through common medical methods. The writer of 1 Timothy suggested wine to soothe Timothy's stomach (1 Timothy 5:23), and this would have been nothing surprising at the time. James, a leader of the church in Jerusalem, told believers to call on the elders in times of illness (James 5:14). Today we largely use James's advice to anoint the sick with oil in a ceremonial way, but at the time it was common Greek medical practice to anoint someone and expect it to help. Our view of specific practices might be different in the twenty-first century, but we can still take to heart the principle that God is able and willing to bring healing through non-miraculous techniques.

By the fourth century, the Christian faith had spread around the Roman Empire. Tradition suggests that Helena, the mother of the emperor Constantine, was the first to open a hospital specifically to care for the poor. The ancient world never had a system to care for the sick who were poor until Christians offered hospitals. Julian was a fourth-century Roman emperor who did not have much use for Christians, and thus became known as Julian the Apostate. Yet even Julian saw what happened when Christians cared for the poor. He wrote, "Now we can see what it is that makes those Christians such powerful enemies of our gods. It is the brotherly love which they manifest toward the sick and poor, the thoughtful manner in which they care for the dead, and the purity of their own lives."

Centuries earlier, the prophet Isaiah spoke of the Messiah to come as the Prince of Peace. Jesus, the fulfillment of the prophecy, brought the kingdom of God to the here and now. Early Christians formed a community to be God's active healing presence in the world. Jesus's ministry of healing both body and spirit pointed to God's active presence in the world. We are still Jesus's disciples, the body of Christ running after God's priorities in the world together.

What does it look like to have a healing ministry in today's world? This is still the question we must be actively answering as people of faith because this question comes from both our own history and our own sacred texts. The century that we live in does not change the essential question and the call for each one of us to engage with it as a robust experience of our personal discipleship.

For Reflection

1. As you read the opening story about the Beale Street Flipper, what did you find to be most challenging to you personally?

2. The author recounted how a friend from his teenage years reappeared in his life when they were both young doctors. When has someone returned unexpectedly to your life in a way that helped you both engage your callings grounded in faith?

3. The author says there are clinics all around the country caring for the underserved, and most of us are unaware of them. Where is the closest one to you? If you don't know, how can you find out?

THREE

FAITH DURING A PANDEMIC

"The patient in Room 3 has a fever and a cough. Should I test him for COVID-19?" My medical assistant looked at me for guidance.

It was March 2020. The COVID-19 pandemic had just gotten started in the United States. The news was filled with mounting deaths in New York City. Fear had reached Memphis, but the virus was just trickling in.

"Yes, let's do that." I replied calmly and then watched my medical assistant gown up like she was headed to Mars. She entered the exam room and closed the door behind her.

Until then, Church Health had built a bubble around me. My senior leaders had, I think rightly, concluded that, as CEO, I should not be seeing any patients with respiratory illnesses who might have the virus. My age alone put me in a risk category for complications. If I got sick, it would have a terrible effect on our staff morale, and I could possibly be prevented from leading the organization at a critical time. It made sense logically, although shaking off the guilt was hard. It felt like I was shirking my duty. Still, the plan was that I wouldn't see any patients who might be infected. I would stick to broken bones and other acute illnesses. But it wasn't going to be that simple. Patients turned up on my watch in walk-in urgent care, and they needed to see a doctor. So there I was in a moment of decision.

When the medical assistant came out of the room, it was time for me to go in. I paused, feeling my heart rate increase with sudden anxiety. It had been over thirty years since I felt that way before encountering a patient.

Thirty years since I had seen my first patient with AIDS.

In 1988, we had no treatment for AIDS. If you got it, you were going to die. We knew it was mostly transmitted through sexual activity, but concern lingered about the possibility of other ways of passing the virus on through less intimate contact. The uncertainty around the transmission of COVID-19 felt familiar in those distant ways.

Doug had been diagnosed with AIDS six months before I first saw him, although he came to me because of other health issues. Before I entered the exam room to see him for the first time, I sensed my heart racing and for the first time paused before entering the room to see a patient. I forged ahead and opened the door. I sat on the rolling stool and began asking questions the same way I would normally. Doug was a young man in his late twenties with long brown hair and a thin face. It looked like he might have been losing weight. He had a couple of sores on his face that I took to be related to the HIV virus. With an engaging personality, Doug answered my questions with long paragraphs rather than simple yes or no answers. He was funny!

I thought I was acting calmly, as if I had treated hundreds of AIDS patients, but I looked down at my hands and could see them sweating. Apparently I was looking down a lot. As I moved forward with the interview, Doug stopped me midsentence.

"You know, Doc, you can't get it from just talking to me."

I looked up and we made eye contact. "You are my first AIDS patient."

"Well, this is the first time I've had AIDS, so we can go through this together." He made me smile, and my heart slowed down.

Unfortunately, Doug died about a year later due to complications from AIDS, but the lesson he taught me that day rushed back to my mind as I stood ready to enter the room of the man with a fever. The difference now was that I might actually get the COVID-19 virus by rolling my stool close enough to talk to my patient in my usual manner.

This was the first time I saw someone in the clinic while wearing a surgical mask, which is not made to endure a lot of conversation. The mask kept sliding down on my nose, and I kept pushing it back up. I knew better. This was the one thing I shouldn't be doing, but the mask was uncomfortable and I felt unprotected. The reflex to adjust it was strong. As time went on, the fallen mask became a common sight. On this occasion, though, I kept pushing it back up.

I asked my questions while staying at least ten feet away. The patient did have a fever, body aches, and a slight cough—cardinal symptoms of COVID-19. I never approached him to examine him. It was an in-person telehealth visit. I told him that we would also test him for the flu, and he didn't seem all that concerned. My worry was greater than his. I don't think he'd been watching the news nonstop the way I had.

As it turns out, there were still lots of other reasons a person could have a cough and a fever in March 2020. It took five days for the results, and his COVID-19 test was negative, but his flu test was positive. He would get better soon. But for months to come, COVID-19 was the first thought I had with every patient I saw.

Getting Personal

From the first call that went out that the pandemic was on its way to Memphis, Church Health began the transformation of virtually everything we do. Our clinic became Fort Knox to everyone trying to enter. Temperature testing, mask wearing, physical distancing, nonclinical employees working remotely, quarantining for contacts or suspected carriers, telemedicine, and drive-through testing. These all became part of our day-to-day operations. For weeks our senior leadership team met daily to implement new procedures to keep serving our patients and the wider community while mitigating risk the best ways we could.

Still, we could not prevent the virus from stabbing our hearts. For years we have run a subspecialty clinic that we staff with retired volunteers. The best doctors in Memphis keep doing what they were born to do solely out of the love of medicine and the desire to do good. Charlie Safley ran a dermatology clinic for us. Dr. Safley had been the skin doctor for the rich and famous of Memphis for many years. He seemed to know everyone. People just called him "Doc," even his three daughters. He always tried to make other people feel needed. If a group picture was being taken, Charlie would grab the camera so the photographer could be in the picture. He did this once at a party, and only later did Charlie learn that the photographer was a professional who had been hired to take pictures. Charlie just laughed.

Before he retired, Charlie saw our patients in his office regularly. After retiring, he came on site a couple of times a month and could treat dozens of patients with skin issues in a short period of time.

In February 2020, the virus was just beginning to spread in the United States. Charlie and friends had planned to go to Mardi Gras in New Orleans and then take a cruise. His close friend Fred Smith, the founder and CEO of FedEx, tried to talk him out of going, but Charlie thought it was safe to follow through on the experience he'd been looking forward to.

When he got back to Memphis, he started running a fever. Within a couple of days, he developed a cough and became short of breath. Then he was in the hospital and placed on a ventilator. Every day we waited for him to get better. And we waited. His kidneys began to fail. And then we got an email saying Charlie had died. We were all crushed.

Then it turned out he was still very much alive. The email had gone out by mistake.

I called one of Charlie's best friends and said, "Charlie would love to be like Mark Twain and say, 'Rumors of my death are greatly exaggerated.'" We laughed, knowing he would love to tell that story.

But the virus was spreading. Although we were relieved about Charlie, we all watched intently as the daily number of new infections rose. Friends and loved ones *would* die.

Calling the Church

In the middle of these early weeks of reorganizing ourselves to keep taking care of people under new protocols, I knew we were doing the best we could. From my incessant news watching, I also knew we, as a society, struggled to know what the right thing was for us to do. But the people asking and answering that question were all politicians, doctors, and public health experts.

Where was the voice of the faith community?

About the middle of March, I began calling faith leaders who had influence over large numbers of people and offered to provide a platform to bring us together. The Catholic bishop, Episcopal bishop, United Methodist bishop, Church of God in Christ bishop, and senior pastors of very large churches—Black and White, Presbyterian, Disciples of Christ, Southern Baptist—along with Reformed Jewish and Islamic congregations, all agreed to begin meeting regularly to forge a way forward as faith leaders and to speak as one voice on a moral strategy for our community. The group trusted me to provide the health facts and guidance from the public health sector, but they committed to standing together, supporting each other, on a way forward. Memphis is an especially religious city. People listen to faith leaders, so this was not a moment for us to miss.

The most pressing question when we first met was the need to close in-person worship. Although we'd only had two deaths in the county at the time, infections were rising. This was not a decision for which anyone had much time to form church committees and discuss and take congregational votes. The pace and danger of infection and the likelihood of congregations' being hot spots meant that between a particular Sunday and midweek gatherings a few days later, services had to be suspended.

At our first meeting, we gathered in person with about fifteen leaders. Hundreds of other clergy watched a webinar via Zoom. I began by speaking on the science of what we knew about COVID-19 at the time. Every eye was on me, trying to glean thoughts about how to lead people whose faith life centered on the houses of worship each of them were responsible for. The bishops all had congregations in rural areas as well as urban. Large and small. Affluent and very poor. The other senior pastors felt the responsibility for thousands of people as well, and pastors of congregations of every size and denomination were listening in and submitting questions. No cookie-cutter plan would fit every congregation, but we knew we had to act soon to keep God's flock safe. The leaders in the room with me committed to being informed by the data and the science and to not making decisions based on gut feelings, the media, or the desire of congregants to be together to worship God.

Bishop David Talley had recently become the Catholic bishop of West Tennessee. He had gotten off on a good foot, but congregations in the diocese were still just getting to know him. He faced the unenviable choice of suspending the obligation of every Catholic—participation in the Mass. "This is fundamental to who we are as Catholics." We could all feel his pressure.

Stacey Spencer, senior pastor of New Directions Christian Church, admitted, "It took a paradigm shift for me to say that as a faith leader I am being more responsible for my people by not meeting. The church is not the building." Around the table others agreed, and the churches of Memphis suspended in-person worship.

Then came the challenges of continuing to be the church while the buildings were closed. Some of the larger congregations were better positioned to weather the disruptions to their normal procedures. They were already streaming services and receiving monetary contributions online. Their congregations were made up of people who were digitally plugged in. But smaller congregations, many made up of less affluent members, depended on meeting together to maintain connections—and budgets. How would the smaller congregations remain financially viable without offerings, keeping the bills and salaries paid when they didn't even know how long it would be before they could gather again?

Then there was the question of how to serve the needs of the community without being physically in contact. Programs like food pantries or soup kitchens, for instance, faced new challenges. What about people who depended on rides to the pharmacy or the doctor? What about older members who needed people checking on them from time to time? These weren't ministries that could simply go on indefinite hiatus without affecting people's well-being in ways that people of faith could just let go and still claim to love their neighbors—not when tens of thousands more were losing their jobs and needs were increasing.

Eventually it would be time to consider whether it was right to reopen churches. Even if the state and local governments said we *could*, did that mean we *should*?

Through all of this was the larger concern, the more important in my mind, of speaking to the broader community beyond our local congregations about what was *right* in a society that was falling apart.

To help with the decision-making, the Church Health staff set up a Facebook page called "Memphis Clergy COVID-19 Response." It was not a very creative title, but it served us well. Our staff organized webinars on maintaining giving, creating virtual worship experiences, hunger-justice ministries, spirituality in children, ministering to the ministers, advanced care directives, virtual funerals, and guidelines for reopening. Hundreds of clergy had access to every topic. We turned notes into downloadable resources that went out to a dedicated email list of clergy. We posted the webinars on the Facebook page and on our website for people to view later. The Facebook page opened connections for sharing resources, discussion topics, cross-training, and moments of prayer. Larger congregations shared know-how and ideas with smaller ones. We also regularly updated the guidelines from the CDC, federal and state government, and the local health department on matters of social distancing and in-person worship. This included posting the grim reports from France, Utah, Arkansas, and other locations that showed that disregard of physical distancing and wearing masks in churches that decided to have in-person worship, over and over, resulted in the spread of the disease and death.

At the end of March, Tim Russell, an associate pastor of Second Presbyterian Church, "2PC," tested positive for the virus. 2PC is an affluent, three-thousand-member congregation that began the pandemic continuing to have in-person worship for those who chose to attend. That all turned on a dime when their beloved pastor got sick, seemed to be improving in the hospital, then abruptly died. In the last week of March, Memphis experienced its first three deaths from COVID-19. Reverend Russell was one of them. Suddenly, most of the faith-community leadership focused completely on its responsibility to keep members safe.

Soon after Tim's death, Eli Morris, the associate pastor of Hope Presbyterian, an even larger church, tested positive. The senior pastor of the church, Rufus Smith, rose to become a leader in the wider church's response. Rufus was one of the first I'd asked to join the group of clergy to speak together on how people of faith should respond.

Those weeks were hard sledding.

This experience of coming to terms with COVID-19, partly through the loss and illness of some of their own, deepened the clergy's understanding of the link between health and faith. Health-care ministry was no longer a feel-good show of having a nurse take blood pressures on Sunday morning during the coffee hour, holding a health fair once a year, or making weak attempts to improve congregational meals by serving less fat and more vegetables. What was now clear was that our bodies and our spirits are one. The physical nature of our existence is critical to who we are, and our ability to respond to God's love is not just a spiritual exercise. Congregations exist to help people experience the fullness of God's love, and that can happen only if we are physically able to respond to the reality around us. Blatant disregard of the physical nature of our created status will disrupt in profound ways the corporate nature of the meaning of the church. The concept of the body of Christ began to take on new meaning.

Our clergy were now very much listening.

Finding New Paths

In the meantime, the disruptive nature of COVID-19 led Church Health to completely rework the way we cared for our patients. For years, we had talked about offering telehealth. Now we were doing it every day with as many patients as possible. Sadly, many low-income people saw telehealth as not "real health care." They regarded it as a cheap substitute for an encounter with the doctor. That the president of the bank would prefer not having to go to a doctor's office made no difference. It was an uphill challenge that we continue to fight.

As the pandemic unfolded, the frequency of COVID-19-positive patients became less frightening—at least to me, although not to our nonmedical staff. We had one then two staff members test positive. Others were reluctant to come to work even when their jobs put them at little risk. While we had as many as possible work from home, fear became a powerful driving force that could not just be wished away.

And then the news came about Dr. Safley. This time the heartbreaking email that he had died was not a mistake.

There was no funeral. No in-person way to tell stories about Doc. No way for grateful patients to express gratitude. We just had to move on. It all seemed wrong.

The people the virus affected the most were those who were always most vulnerable. The demographics stirred the pot when it became clear that people of color were disproportionately infected. The virus, however, had no regard for race or country of origin. What it did do is prey on those who couldn't protect themselves, people who had no choice but to go to work even when there were no means of protection for them.

On a Sunday night, I was watching *60 Minutes*, the CBS newsmagazine show. They aired a segment on how people in the meatpacking industry were being disproportionately infected with COVID-19. I was only halfway paying attention when the voice from the TV said, "The hardest hit community in Texas is a small town known as Cactus."

I began watching intently. Cactus was where Dr. Stephanie Diehlmann was located, working in the Church of the Nazarene's clinic The Well. Even though I have never been to Cactus, their suffering seemed close to home because I knew Steph.

I reached out the next morning to Steph. I didn't hear back for a couple of days, but finally we were able to talk. She calmly began, "We are only a county of 20,000 people, but we have five hundred cases so far." The virus had to be far more widespread than just the five hundred cases that had been detected.

She went on. "Almost everyone works in the meatpacking plant. They have tried, but there is only so much they can do. The governor has said they can't shut down. The workers are considered essential, so they keep going because they have to get paid."

I felt helpless talking to her, but she remained upbeat. "Our medical teams are working really well together. We know God will watch over us. This is why we are here." What great courage and faith.

Across the country similar scenarios have played out. The poor in every community were the largest group becoming infected. How were families with seven or eight people living in a two-bedroom apartment supposed to socially distance? Whether in Cactus, Atlanta, Memphis, or so many other cities, people in impoverished neighborhoods and in communities of color found themselves disproportionately choosing between risking infection or risking eviction. As one of our local pastors said of his Hispanic congregation, it wasn't that they wanted to break the public health guidelines, but they had to go to work to pay rent and eat.

And then vicious rumors emerged. Despite the facts, it became a common belief in some communities that Blacks couldn't get the disease and that face masks and testing actually spread the virus. As we began setting up drive-through testing sites in underserved neighborhoods, it was clear that the first task was to convince people that testing was important and could keep them safe. Our best communicators for this were pastors. And so we continued to reach out through our Facebook page, our webinars, TV, radio, and every type of social media we could touch so that the voice of the church could speak with faith about the health of the community.

It was heartwarming to see the way laypeople began doing all they could to make a difference. In churches, people sewed face masks in every way you can conceive. Small businesses began making face shields and donating to us and other frontline workers. An affluent dressmaking shop made designer face masks for a variety of frontline medical clinics. The link between faith and health was being forged in tangible ways no one could have foreseen.

The Story in Numbers

When the COVID-19 pandemic began, more than half of US workers shifted to working from home. Those who continued to work their normal jobs by showing up at workplaces in person were people deemed "essential workers." We all learned that phrase, but who were these people and what did their risk tell us about health-care disparities? We heard every day about the risks that health-care workers and first responders took while working in direct contact with patients who were, or could be, infected with the COVID-19 virus. At least in the beginning, we heard much less about the millions of low-wage workers who were deemed essential and what that meant for their health. The half of us who could shift to working from home nevertheless depended on people who couldn't. Someone had to keep the grocery store shelves stocked, deliver food we weren't willing to go out to buy ourselves, make sure we could get our prescriptions, fulfill the mammoth amount of online orders that took over retail shopping, and try to keep the economy going at some basic level.

The Coronavirus Aid, Relief, and Economic Security (CARES) Act passed in March 2020 provided funding for up to two weeks of paid days for illness, quarantining, or caring for a family member with COVID-19. But the legislation included exemptions for large businesses with more than five hundred employees. People working in grocery store chains, for instance, who could be exposed to the virus every time they went to work, did not have paid-leave protection. People working in agricultural companies and the meatpacking industry were essential because they kept the country fed, but they were also exempted from paid sick leave. In the meatpacking industry alone, this required workers to continue to work in crowded, poorly ventilated spaces. Forty-four percent of all meatpackers are Latinx, and 80 percent of all agricultural workers speak only Spanish. The end result is that at the height of the pandemic, according to the CDC, the hospitalization rate of the Latinx population with COVID-19 was 320 per 100,000 population compared to 116 per 100,000 for Whites. In California, where 39 percent of the population is Latinx, they accounted for 60.6 percent of the COVID-19 cases and 48.5 percent of deaths six months into the pandemic. Studies suggested that risk factors among the Latinx population for infection included crowded households, a lack of English proficiency, being young, and working in jobs classified as essential, such as meatpacking and food service. Faced with the suggestion that it would be safer for themselves and their families not to work in the unsafe conditions of many of their jobs, the common response is that they have to work. "Tengo que trabajar."[1] Many people would say the same thing in a lot of other languages, including English.

Within the first six months of the pandemic, data from multiple sources at federal, state, and local levels quickly showed that people of color experienced a greater burden of both cases, hospitalizations, and deaths from COVID-19. This was true in more than thirty states out of the forty-four that reported data. People of color faced a greater economic toll as well. These realities were widespread across the country. Disparities related to COVID-19 brought to light unjust disparities tied up in social, economic, and health inequities that existed prior to the pandemic.[2]

Across the board, inequalities quickly emerged in historically disadvantaged communities. A study out of the Department of Sociology of Indiana University about the vulnerability of certain populations to the impact of the pandemic found that Black adults were three times more likely to experience food insecurity, be laid off from their jobs, or become unemployed in the long term than were White residents in the areas they studied. The same was true for women and younger adults. Groups that were already experiencing disadvantages now took the biggest hits because of economy closures and health risks. The pandemic disproportionately affected historically disadvantaged groups, leading to even greater inequity. We've known for a long time that disease and death rates fall disproportionately along racial and disadvantaged lines. Now the pandemic has shown us just how quickly—practically instantly—these precariously situated groups experienced a negative impact on their physical and financial well-being that other groups were able to navigate and weather with less startling statistics.[3]

People in rural areas have been another group to watch. The forty-six million Americans who live in rural counties have faced challenges people in urban areas may be less familiar with in general—health and socioeconomic disparities that heightened the risk of contracting COVID-19, the distance to the nearest hospital or to a hospital that supports a higher level of care, the poverty rate, obstacles to mental health services in counties that may not have a single psychiatrist.⁴ These conditions were true before the pandemic, and I suspect they will be true after the pandemic, but COVID-19 certainly cast a floodlight on the truth.

The Push to Open

Only a few months into the pandemic, the push to reopen churches began. President Trump declared that churches were essential and should open "now." But it wasn't that simple. If a church was to open with 25 percent or 50 percent capacity, how exactly was that to happen? Was the pastor to choose who got to come to church or who got to partake of communion? Filling the pews was surely unsafe. The best information at the time made clear that one of the greatest risks of the spread of COVID-19 in churches was singing, so how were we to make a joyful noise without risking the people sitting near us?

These challenges persisted. The world has changed, and how faith communities are reimagining themselves is an ongoing process. Hopefully we have learned that following the original call to discipleship remains our way forward. "Love your neighbor" is not just a plaque on the church wall. To follow Jesus, the Bible calls us to preach, to teach, and to heal. Engaging in a healing ministry has always been a part of who we are as Christians and people of faith. Somewhere along the way, we lost our line of vison to seeing who Jesus is.

Even the biggest skeptics of who Jesus is do not doubt that he was a healer in the first-century world of Galilee. It is also certain that the growth of the church in the first three centuries AD was greatly influenced by Christians who risked their own lives during plagues throughout the Roman world because they believed that's what Jesus would have done. A healing ministry is central to what it means to follow Jesus.

To us, a pandemic is a new experience, but of course history tells us it is not new. Even if we only scan the centuries since Jesus—the life of the Christian church—we see that the Plague of Cyprian, the bishop of Carthage in the third century, killed a million people in two decades. In some accounts, two thousand people a day were dying in Rome. Three centuries later, the Plague of Justinian, named for the Roman emperor in Constantinople, killed thirty to fifty million. In the Middle Ages, the Black Death took two hundred million lives and smallpox fifty-six million. In more recent centuries, we battled cholera, yellow fever, and scarlet fever. We only have to look back over the last hundred years to see the 1918–1920 influenza pandemic (estimated to have killed forty to fifty million worldwide), polio, HIV/AIDS, and H1N1 just a few years ago. Many of these pandemics were staggering in worldwide impact, which included fallen economies.

All of these have been opportunities for people of faith to embrace healing ministry, even at personal risk, and in fact we have many historical examples of Jesus's followers doing so, from caring for the poor when no one else would, to opening the first hospitals, to staying behind when others distanced themselves from the disease by fleeing cities to the countryside, to the preacher Cotton Mather advocating for inoculations and experimenting on himself. When we ask ourselves now what we can do to serve the underserved in a pandemic, and afterward, we stand in a long tradition.

In Memphis, in the days after Martin Luther King Jr. was assassinated in 1968, the clergy of the city came together to ask, Where do we go from here and can we do it together? The result was the creation of MIFA, the Metropolitan Interfaith Association. This is a large multiservice social agency that has existed in Memphis for over fifty years. The Memphis Food Bank grew out of MIFA and continues to have the same spirit, collaborating with congregations and nonprofits to make sure the rising numbers of food-insecure people during the pandemic were fed. During COVID-19, in the drive-through testing sites Church Health ran, everyone seeking a test was also offered a trunk full of groceries from Memphis Food Bank if they needed food. This was a tangible way to show that Dr. King's vision of justice is still very much alive.

COVID-19 focused an unexpected lens on faith and health. The question for us now is whether we take this crisis and create a new response to the pain and suffering of the world. We have shown that we can coalesce around a tragedy, but can we carry on with what we have learned when things are again "normal"?

I'm convinced that we can.

George Robertson, senior pastor at Second Presbyterian Church, where Tim Russell served, says the pandemic will leave a holistic impact. "Not only has the virus made people physically sick, but fear of the virus and quarantining has made them emotionally and spiritually sick. My care for people has had to involve a team approach with medical providers, behavioral health experts, social workers, educators, financial counselors, and relational experts. The whole person has been attacked with illness, and the whole person bearing in a multifaceted way the image of God has to be approached with gospel-centered love."

Micah Greenstein, senior rabbi at Temple Israel, says the lasting experiences of the pandemic have "reinforced that it is the poor and people of color who continue to pay the most in health deficits, COVID-19 infections, mental illness, and dislocation from whatever 'normal' was, is, or ever will be."

Both of these colleagues, who have been in the trenches with me, are right.

COVID-19 tore the fabric of our world, our churches, and our lives apart. Returning to how it had "always been" is never going to happen. In the past when great tragedy struck the world or the church, people of faith responded with new insight and fresh vision. Re-embracing the healing ministry of the church is one of the great opportunities we now have before us. It isn't an option to close our eyes to the link we know exists between body and spirit. Jesus healed the man born blind in John's Gospel, and when the man for the first time saw the many ways that God loves the world, he was fully ready to follow Jesus. We too must be healed of our blindness. When we are, we will see the full richness of the calling to ministry for the underserved that God has set before us.

The experience of being the church in the midst of a pandemic opened our eyes to yearning for hope. Uncertainty rolled like waves that never let us catch our breath. Health and economic anxiety mounted. We couldn't even gather to hug each other through it. Even the people who prematurely said they were "done" with staying home or "over" having to wear a mask were in their own way searching for hope that the uncertainty would end and we would know the end of the story.

The pandemic brought to light many inequities in our life as a nation—access to health care if you got COVID-19, paid time off if you needed to quarantine because you were exposed, the ability to be tested, the kinds of jobs that were supported by unemployment benefits, what happens when millions of people suddenly lose their employer health insurance. We wrestled to respond. We weren't flawless by any stretch, but there was a sense that the virus shouldn't be the dividing line. Many issues have been dividing lines for many years that shouldn't be. What are we going to do about them now that the pandemic made this truth so crystal clear to us?

Can we as people of faith pick up that thread and carry it forward with a broader view of equity in health care because the pandemic has given us a lens we didn't expect?

I said to our staff on nearly a daily basis while we were finding our way through the early months of the pandemic that we are not alone. God is with us. That is hope. And when the church embraces a healing ministry, we offer healing hope during a pandemic and beyond.

For Reflection

1. What were your own emotions at the beginning of the COVID-19 pandemic? Did your feelings change as the outbreak in your area settled in? How about after the pandemic raged on, yet the economy and society opened up?
2. Do trying times make it harder for you to find your spiritual center or do you dig in deeper when challenges arise? What experiences do you think form your reactions?
3. Has the church been a place of refuge for you during hard times or a place where it's hard to let people know times are hard? Why do you think this is?

FOUR

WHY DO THOSE PILLS COST SO MUCH?

"Her husband is the problem." Kim was unequivocal, adamant about the situation. "Uh-huh, he lets her do all the work. He should be working three jobs, but it all falls to her."

Kim Simmons was the first employee I ever hired for Church Health—if you don't count the person I hired to work at the front desk and then figured out in the first two hours of her shift that she was actively schizophrenic and hallucinating. I had to let her go.

I then turned to the Memphis Medical Society, which ran a temporary service for office staff. They sent me Kim. She was in her late twenties with long black hair piled up high. She had been working as needed in the emergency room at Baptist Memorial Hospital but wanted a full-time job. I told her what we were about, and she said, "That's just what I need." We are still working together. She has had more positions than I can count. These days she works in compliance to help all our providers stay credentialed as well as wrangling with any insurance we accept, which we do for limited reasons. It is a thankless job, but Kim does it with grace. There is almost no one whom I respect more or whose judgment I trust more than Kim's. She is a rock.

I was there when Kim got married to Tony a couple of years after she started working at the front desk. I was also there when she had her only child, Gabriel, and watched as Gabriel grew up. She became a cheerleader and then went off to college.

Along the way, I would run into Kim's mom and dad from time to time. I always sang her praises to her parents because I knew they liked to hear it. Her father, Charles, is only a few years older than I am. He is a big man with a deep voice who loves his baby girl. We get along great.

Then a couple of years ago, Charles's health started to fade. He had a stroke and began to have dementia. When he was struggling the most, Kim came to work every day and did what she was asked to do, but I could tell it was weighing on her. It was even harder on her mom. Then one day, Kim asked me for a favor. Kim never asks me for a favor.

"We've found this woman who is really good with Daddy," Kim said. "He likes her, and she takes good care of him. But she has problems, and she doesn't have health insurance. Do you think you can see her?"

"Kim, of course I will see her." I was surprised she felt like she needed to ask. "Just make her an appointment."

"She doesn't live in Memphis. She lives in Tunica."

Kim told me this because we have a rule that patients have to live in Shelby County, which includes Memphis, in order to be a regular patient. I made that rule years ago when I first saw a twelve-year-old girl with anorexia nervosa. She was trying to die. At twelve, she weighed no more than sixty pounds. She was painful to look at. Nothing I could say to her made any difference. Her body image was that she was fat and needed to lose weight. The big challenge was that she and her family lived in Jackson, Mississippi, a four-hour drive from Memphis. Still, I couldn't just walk away. I made phone call after phone call to get her admitted to a psychiatric hospital that treated eating disorders. Eventually she got better, but I used up a lot of favors and resources. I felt like God had put her in front of me, and I couldn't wash my hands of her, but our whole ministry is a great exercise in scarce resources. We have to draw a line somewhere. Driving four hours to see us wasn't tenable, and neither was using up favors for someone that far outside our community. I made the decision that patients need to live in Shelby County.

However, I have always said, "We have guidelines not rules." Because I made up that Shelby County rule, I can break it whenever I want. I know that is cavalier and not something we can do every time, but when God is speaking we must listen.

I told Kim I could see her father's caregiver through our walk-in clinic in order to understand the problem, and then I would make a long-term plan.

Kim replied, "Thank you, Jesus."

She knew where our ability to help comes from, so I agreed with her. "Yes, thank Jesus if we can make a difference."

Two days later I met Bobbie in the clinic. She wasn't exactly what I anticipated. She was in her late forties, overweight, and had a hard edge. With unkempt clothes and uncombed hair, she sat in the chair skeptical of everything I said. It seemed clear that she had not always had good experiences with doctors.

I began in my usual way. After introducing myself I asked, "What can I do to help you?"

She answered, "I doubt anything."

Not a good way to start.

She continued, "I'm out of all of my medicine. I can't afford them." I looked over on the counter where she had laid at least ten drugs. My first thought was, Nobody needs this many drugs. Usually, I am right about that. Few people on ten drugs need all of them.

As I made my way down the list, I could tell she had a boatload of problems. After telling me all her aches and pains she ended with, "They tell me I have lupus."

I was skeptical, but the more we talked, the more I began to think she might really have lupus, a form of arthritis where the body makes antibodies against itself. It effectively attacks healthy tissues, thinking the body's own substance is foreign and harmful. The result is a person's joints and other important organs are in a self-destructive free fall.

In the past, medical treatments for lupus were mostly ineffective. Today, the biologic category of drugs constantly advertised on TV actually stop the disease from progressing and at times even reverse its progress. The challenge is that the costs of the medicine can run into thousands of dollars—every week.

"My doctor tried to give me those things in Chicago," Bobbie said. "He gave me a couple of shots in his office and it seemed to help. Then he gave me a prescription. How was I to afford that?"

I knew what she meant. The commercials give people hope without mentioning the expense. In some cases, though, we have been able to get the drugs through a patient assistance program, or PAP. It might be possible we could get the medicine for free, but Bobbie would have to work with us to fill out all the forms.

Still, her problems went beyond the cost of the lupus drugs. She had diabetes, requiring insulin, and extremely high blood pressure. On top of that, she clearly had family problems, which Kim had pointed out.

"I had to leave Chicago because my medicine was so expensive. I couldn't afford our rent. My mom is down here, so I hoped we could make it work back in Mississippi." Bobbie sighed. "But of course, it's no better here."

She was living in Tunica, Mississippi, near the casinos. Her husband made $10 an hour with no benefits working as a janitor. They had moved in with her mom, who needed Bobbie to help in a variety of ways. Bobbie got a job as a certified nursing assistant (CNA) at a nursing home where Kim's sister, Lauren, is the administrator. She worked forty hours a week. Because she was a hard worker and caught Lauren's eye, Lauren asked if Bobbie wanted a second job helping care for Kim and Lauren's father in the family home. Bobbie jumped at the chance.

From my observation, I just couldn't see Bobbie being a good caregiver. I was dead wrong. "Oh, honey, she is so good to my daddy and my momma," Kim said. "She does everything. She works Monday, Tuesday, and Wednesday from seven till nine at night and on Saturday from nine to nine."

I began to see why Bobbie looked tired and worn out when I met her in the clinic.

Kim kept on. "We love her. Sometimes when she's at my mom's house she goes in the back to take a nap. We are trying to figure out how she might be able to rent Tony's mom's house." Again Kim pointed out that Bobbie's husband is less than helpful. "He is the one who should be working three jobs, but I think it has always been on her. Working at Sam's Town for $10 an hour is just wrong." Kim was clear where she stood.

I drew Bobbie's blood to confirm that she did indeed have lupus.

Because of knowing how much Bobbie mattered to Kim, I did my best to encourage her to take advantage of everything we offer. Help with getting the medicine, one of the counselors, our physical therapist, a dietician, a dentist. She could use almost everything we offer, and the cost would be minimal.

As we were about to draw her blood I told her, "I am sure we can help you have less pain."

She looked away. "I don't have the money."

She just couldn't hear what I was offering. Maybe because I am an old White guy. Maybe because she can't believe anyone would want to help her.

"Let's get the blood test results, and then when you come back in two weeks we can work on the bigger plan."

"Whatever." She remained looking down.

The blood test indicated that there was active inflammation, which meant her joints were bound to be hurting. The new biologic drugs would most likely help both the pain and the progression of the disease.

Two weeks went by. I stopped by Kim's office and asked, "Do you know why Bobbie didn't come back for her appointment?"

"She just has too many things going against her," Kim said. "We keep trying to help her. She is so good to my daddy, but she has one problem after the other. Maybe if we can get her to move into Tony's mother's home she will come back. I don't know." Kim was clearly frustrated. But she couldn't make Bobbie take the help we were offering.

The constant drumming of being beaten down can prevent people from seeing hope when it is right before them. It makes no sense unless you have had hope ripped away from you time and again. I truly don't know what that is like. But few things can be so horrid.

I reassured Kim that when the time came, I would be ready to see Bobbie, or if she would rather see one of the other doctors, I would make that happen too.

"No, Scott, I want her to see you. She needs to see you." Kim made me feel like I hadn't totally failed. At least I know what we need to do if Bobbie does come back. I will be ready.

The Price Is Not Right

John's right wrist was red and swollen and terribly painful. I could tell he was very uncomfortable. In his mid-fifties and with hair gray, he works as a painter and needs his wrist to make enough money to care for his family. And I could tell he had always worked as a laborer. His clothes were dotted with paint, his skin was weathered. He is not a big man, but he is strong, and he was not one to come to the doctor unless he felt desperate.

John had not fallen or done anything to hurt his wrist. I couldn't see any source of infection, which left me with the most obvious cause of his problem—he had gout.

Gout is a form of arthritis caused by a substance that naturally occurs in the blood called uric acid. When the body makes too much uric acid, crystals can form and then settle in a joint, which leads to extreme pain. The most common place for this to occur is the big toe, but it can happen in any joint. I have practiced medicine long enough to recognize the symptoms.

I was sure John had gout, and I was also sure John would not be able to afford the most effective medicine to relieve his pain—colchicine. Colchicine is a remarkable drug. Within a few hours of beginning to take the medicine, a patient can experience complete relief from pain. When I first started to practice medicine, it was incredibly rewarding to prescribe colchicine for a person with gout.

Someone I saw in the morning would call me back in the afternoon to tell me what a great doctor I am. Several friends over the years concluded the same when I gave them a prescription for colchicine. It truly can seem like a miracle drug.

And then on July 20, 2009, all of that changed.

An Egyptian papyrus from 1500 BC describes the use of the substance colchicine for the treatment of rheumatism. It was first used for the treatment of gout in the first century AD. In 550 it appears as "hermodactyl" in an early list of drugs. It is listed in the *London Pharmacopoeia of 1618*. It was brought to the United States by Benjamin Franklin, who made fun of his gout in writings while he was the ambassador to France. In 1833 the purified ingredient was isolated and named colchicine. Ever since, physicians in the United States have used it readily when they recognize the acute pain of gout.

In 2006, the US Food and Drug Administration began the Unapproved Drug Initiative. This was intended to regulate drugs that had not been proven to be effective and required pharmaceutical companies to go through extensive testing to prove a drug's effectiveness. As it happens, no one had ever conducted double-blind controlled studies to demonstrate that colchicine actually works, although Benjamin Franklin could have told you that it does. So URL Pharma did a controlled study on 185 patients and received a patent to market colchicine under the brand name Colcrys.

Patent in hand, the company then sued to have all generic forms being sold by other pharmaceutical companies removed from the market. They were successful.

Overnight, the cost of colchicine went from $0.09 per pill to $4.85, an almost 2,000 percent increase. Obviously this put colchicine out of the reach of most low-income, uninsured patients who suffered from gout. In 2012, URL Pharma was acquired by Takeda for $800 million, and the primary value of the company was the exclusivity of the gout medication. The patent is in place until 2029.

John was one of the patients left behind by the increase in the price of this ancient medication for gout pain. I had to find another way to treat John's pain. My go-to plan these days is to use prednisone, an anti-inflammatory steroid that has many potential side effects. While it is inexpensive, in addition to its side effects, it takes several days to begin to work. This meant that I also prescribed John narcotics to deal with his pain more immediately until the prednisone could begin to work. I didn't even mention colchicine to him. Maybe I should have let him choose whether he wanted to endure the pain for a few more days or spend money he didn't have for quicker relief. I was torn, but in the end I just wrote the prescriptions for prednisone and the narcotic.

It was a Friday when I saw him. On Sunday I called his house to see how he was doing. His daughter answered the phone. "My daddy is so much better. Thank you for helping him."

I was relieved that he had begun to have relief sooner than I expected. Only two days. "Make sure he comes to see me this week so we can try and prevent him from going through this again." She was glad to pass on my message.

Every time I treat a patient with gout, I feel my blood boiling about what happened with this centuries-old drug. How can a drug company claim to own something that has been known to be effective for centuries and in doing so take away from the poor a truly miraculous drug? But that is what happened. A few people complained, but most people felt that URL Pharma had just followed the rules and were smarter than everyone else

to see the opportunity. There was no consideration of morality. No sermon
was ever preached on the subject. People tried to find a way to help poor
people afford the cost rather than ask, Why has the cost gone up exponen-
tially? One more time, profits from medicine outweigh caring for those
who are least among us.

Following the Money

What good is a brilliant diagnosis if the patient can't afford the treatment?
I have had to deal with this reality for over thirty years. While I don't think
that pharmaceuticals can solve all health-care problems, they are an important part of modern medicine, and their costs have skyrocketed in the
last three decades.

When I began Church Health in 1987, I had few options for getting pharmaceutical medicines to our patients. Generic drugs were not as common
as they are today, and the internet didn't exist as a means to find cheap
drugs. The one source that was fairly easy to come by was drug samples
delivered almost daily by pharmaceutical reps. Drug reps would appear at
the clinic's front desk asking to see the doctor. If I was willing to give the
rep a few minutes of my time to hear about new products, the rep would
leave samples of the drug that I could give to patients. The samples would
usually have anywhere from a few days' to a week's supply in a box.

Usually, a rep would leave a handful of sample packages for one doctor,
but as I was readily willing to talk to any rep who showed up, some of them
started to leave samples in large quantities. As the reps came to understand the mission of Church Health, a number of them were moved to be
even more generous. The problem was that some of the most generous-
minded reps carried the least useful medicines. Some days I would get
a large supply of a drug I rarely used. I might also be left with drugs that
needed a prescription but were just a glorified version of a cold medicine
that anyone can buy over the counter. For the most part, I was not looking
for exotic medications for cancer or rare diseases but drugs that would be
quite inexpensive for most people who have insurance, such as medicine
to control cholesterol or hypertension or diabetes.

The Memphis Medical Representatives Association took us on as a
charity they supported. The group met on a monthly basis and often in-

vited me to speak to them. Most importantly, they created a golf tournament where the proceeds benefited Church Health. The pharmaceutical reps invited doctors they called on to play for free, and the companies they represented would make a donation. This helped us significantly in caring for patients when we first began.

As I had more opportunities to tell our story, especially in faith communities, groups would want to volunteer to help. Early on, a group of women delivered boxes of rolled-up bandages made from old sheets. Each was tied with a nice bow. It looked like something out of *Gone with the Wind*. I knew I had to find a way for people to volunteer, and having them help with the drugs seemed an easy solution.

Laws around pharmaceuticals from the Food and Drug Administration have always been strict. Historically, the FDA worried about the efficacy and manufacture of drugs, but in 1982 that all changed. In a suburb of Chicago, five people died over a three-day period after being poisoned with potassium cyanide. Investigators quickly discovered that the cyanide had been inserted into capsules containing Tylenol. Mass hysteria consumed the country while millions of bottles of Tylenol and other over-the-counter medicines were destroyed. The laws around repurposing drugs tightened. Once a bottle was opened it could not be sold or even given away to another patient. As a result, billions of dollars of medicines were literally flushed down the toilet.

Even years after this event, people throughout the city didn't understand the new laws, so they continued to drop off at our door boxes of medicine they hoped we could use for our patients. Sadly, we could not use them. Either staff or volunteers were needed to find a safe way to destroy the donations.

What remained legal, however, was our finding creative ways to acquire more and more sample meds. As time went on, our pharmaceutical rep friends would empty out their store closets and deliver large quantities of drugs to us. In addition, we would ask other doctors to give us their samples rather than use them for patients who had health insurance and prescription drug plans. Taking full advantage of this led to our engaging dozens of "little old ladies doing drugs" and sending young future doctors and retired business executives on "drug runs."

Since the sample boxes rarely held more than one week's supply of pills, we needed to find a way to reduce the bulk so that patients didn't have to go home with two garbage sacks of mostly cardboard when they left the clinic with three months' worth of medicine.

Removing pills from their sample bubble packages was now illegal, so we began to condense medicine with the help of volunteers. Syl Marks and her friends became faithful pill packers. Syl was the daughter of Elias Goldsmith, who started the iconic department store in Memphis known as Goldsmith's. Syl was in her early seventies when I first met her, and she asked to become a volunteer. Syl was no more than four foot ten, but she was an irresistible force. She had a way of holding her hands almost as though she was praying and would tilt her head to the right. Her black hair was pulled back, and she was always dressed immaculately. She would begin, "Scott, you are such an important part of Memphis." I learned to wait for the next line, which was usually, "I need you to do me a little favor." It was never a little anything, but it was impossible to say no.

Syl used that ploy on the Sisterhood of Temple Israel, and before I knew it a faithful group of older Jewish women sat around a conference table in our original building once a month. For hours they would cram as many cards of sample pills as possible into one cardboard manufacturer's box. Each box could now hold a month or more of medicine rather than just a few pills. It was tedious but rewarding work for the women, and the patients would benefit.

As the process became more efficient, we were always looking to acquire more sample medicine. Many doctors in town agreed to give us their samples but required us to pick them up from their offices. In time, we began hiring clinic assistants to do the work. These were very bright recent college graduates who were taking a year off of study but who wanted to go to medical school. During their gap year they would acquire clinical experience working for us. Overseeing the sample-medicine program became a full-time job for several of them every year.

Shane, on one occasion, was making a "drug run," picking up samples from multiple doctors' offices. Shane had long hair and was wearing scrubs. He was driving an old beat-up car when he didn't see an oncoming car and had a wreck on a major street. His vehicle was filled with sample medicines, mostly to treat blood pressure and diabetes. The pills flew all over the road. This was before cell phones, so Shane was left alone to explain his way out of the situation when the police arrived.

Shane is now a cardiologist, but I know that day was one of the most hair-raising experiences he has ever had in medicine. Thankfully he was not carrying any controlled substances. In today's world, with the opioid epidemic, it is hard to believe that hydrocodone and Xanax were once readily given out as samples. Pharmaceutical reps used to leave as many narcotics samples as they did blood pressure pills.

Around 2000, the large pharmaceutical companies began to feel increased pressure as a result of the rising cost of drugs and the reality that medicines that had once been affordable for the working uninsured were now ten times as expensive. In response, pharmaceutical companies began programs that allowed patients to receive their drugs for free "if they qualified." Each company developed their own qualifications and their own forms. It was time-consuming for patients to fill out the forms, but it seemed to be worth it.

In 2002, the pharmaceutical companies created the patient assistance program, an organization that sought to work together within the industry to provide patients drugs for free and stave off pressure from Washington. They held a conference in Princeton, New Jersey, and invited me to speak. The people gathered were mostly new in their positions and had little power in the companies, but some of them sincerely wanted to do good.

I tried my best to talk to as many company reps as possible. I made the most headway with the person representing AstraZeneca, a large company that had just recently started promoting "the purple pill," Prilosec, used for heartburn and other stomach issues. Their person was Cynthia, a woman with blond hair in her mid-forties and dressed in a business suit like everyone else. Kind but guarded, she nevertheless seemed open and curious about the work we do. I began my pitch to her and she listened.

"Did you know that of the people who are working and uninsured today, 30 percent of them within one to two years will have a job that offers them health insurance? If you give away your chronic-disease medicines today, if they are working, when those people get health insurance, the doctor is highly unlikely to change what they are on. So, by giving away your drugs, you have a 30 percent chance of making a long-term sell within one to two years."

Cynthia listened. She clearly hadn't thought in those terms. She told me she would take what I had said back to her bosses.

I didn't expect much. Several months later, I noticed a change in the ads for Prilosec. At the end of every commercial, there was the statement, "If you cannot afford your medicine, AstraZeneca might be able to help you." I never knew for sure, but I have always wondered if my conversation helped create that statement.

When the conference in Princeton was over, I rode back to the airport in a cab with one of the other speakers. He was the head of a division of the Health Resources and Services Administration within the federal department of Health and Human Services that oversees the pharmaceutical industry. I was most interested in talking to him because he oversaw the 340B drug-pricing program. This is a federal program that buys drugs from pharmaceutical companies at a greatly discounted rate and then allows hospitals and clinics to purchase them at that price for the purpose of distributing the drugs to the disadvantaged. I wanted Church Health to be able to participate in the program, but we have never been allowed to do so. The program is only open to "covered entities," which means a clinic that is funded by the federal government to care for the poor. If a clinic doesn't receive federal dollars for the purpose of purchasing the drugs, then it is not eligible for the program. An organization like Church Health, funded by charitable donations rather than federal tax dollars, has no access to these discounted drugs. That has always struck me as ludicrous.

It was ninety minutes back to the airport. Halfway back I felt sorry for my cab mate. He was nice enough. He wore a dark suit and looked like he worked for the government. He had the air about him I have come to know from people in jobs like his. He was respectful, polite, and willing to listen. He heard me out and even seemed to sympathize with our plight. When I had finished, though, he simply answered, "I don't think I can help you."

That was it.

There was no more to say. The last twenty minutes of the ride were silent. I didn't have another move to make. I was stymied and have been stymied on this issue ever since.

That left us to continue to be creative to find medicine for our patients. We turned our sample program into a cottage industry. We hired more and more recent graduates to work for a year helping acquire and condense our medicines. We had a group of pill packers every morning and every afternoon. We worried about keeping lot numbers and expiration dates logged into a database. When patients with multiple problems left the clinic, they had large boxes of medicine. It was fulfilling but not efficient or sustainable.

And then the pharmaceutical companies stopped supplying samples. Instead, they began giving out coupons that offered a discount—but only for the first few months of starting a drug.

Generic manufacturers, along with large chain drug stores, began offering $4 a month generic medicine. This seems like an incredibly generous offer until you realize the cost of making the medicine can be only a few cents a month. Nevertheless, it was a great help.

Others entered the world of providing pharmaceuticals for low-wage earners and the uninsured. In Memphis, Good Shepherd Pharmacy allowed patients to pay a monthly fee and then they would do much of the work we were doing. It has been a good partnership.

We have also searched for other sources of medicine. Nursing homes throw away billions of dollars of drugs every year, yet it has been illegal for them to redistribute the medicine even though it is packaged in unit doses, meaning in individual doses, so that it can't be tampered with. Oklahoma was the first state to allow nursing homes to redistribute the meds to pharmacies like Good Shepherd. Tennessee has now followed suit.

In the meantime, the cost of new drugs has become unbelievable.

Maxine is a forty-year-old woman who works as a housekeeper. Two years ago she began having increasing pain in her hands and feet. She put it down to her work until it became harder and harder to get out of bed. Then she came to our clinic. The knuckles of both hands were starting to become deformed, and her hands were warm to the touch. It was clear she had rheumatoid arthritis. I began her on $4 a month medicine to see if it could control the pain. It helped some but not enough to matter.

Next, I started her on methotrexate, a drug used for cancer that can help prevent the disease from advancing. The problem is that it has lots of side effects and doesn't work well for rheumatoid arthritis. I knew Maxine needed a biologic drug that would most likely stop the disease from advancing, but the cost can be over $5,000 a month. There was no way she would ever be able to afford that. Who could?

These drugs are hard to come by through patient assistance programs. Thankfully, our staff persisted. Maxine was started on the drug and almost immediately began having relief. For now, she is better, but can we continue to supply her medicine for the rest of her life? Who is to say?

This is the challenge of providing health care in the name of the church. It is a never-ending challenge of advocacy. And what about patients who don't have someone knowledgeable to advocate for them? People are still caught in the gaps and don't know how to get out on their own. They only know they can't afford the medication that can prevent a stroke or control their blood sugar or manage their pain.

The Story in Numbers

If you know someone with diabetes—and most of us do—then you probably pay attention to stories in the news about the rising costs of insulin. The story is similar to gout medication. Although insulin is not as ancient, we know who discovered it, and it goes beyond relieving pain to saving lives. Yet along with EpiPens, another life-saving medication that has long been affordable and saw giant price increases in recent years for no better reason than because the patent holder knew people would pay higher prices to carry an injection that could save their child's life, the price of insulin has been in the hands of the patent holders.

The original inventors never envisioned what has happened. Frederick Banting and John J. R. MacCloud, who shared the 1923 Nobel Prize in Physiology or Medicine, did not want to be named as patent holders of their discovery of insulin. Banting articulated that to do so would violate his Hippocratic oath. A medical student and a biochemist faced no such dilemma, and their names, Charles Best and James B. Collip, went on the patent application as inventors. However, they also believed that insulin should be made widely available and cost should be no barrier, so for one dollar they transferred all rights of the patent to the governors of the University of Toronto.[1]

Somehow we got from there to where we are now. The major pharmaceutical companies that manufacture insulin would say they have improved on it in the last hundred years, including developing synthetic forms. A variety of types of insulin are available. Not everyone would agree that the differences between them justify the price increases. Is the newer form that costs twenty times as much as an older variety really twenty times better?

And what about the ones that aren't really any different but just cost more than they used to? Insulin can range from $25 to $300 per vial, and some people may need six vials a month.

Colchicine and insulin and the others I've mentioned are only a few medications in the US medication landscape that make a lot of people scratch their heads about why things cost so much. The United States spends an average of $1,229 per person each year on pharmaceuticals, far outpacing other countries of similar economic status. In a 2019 comparison of per capita spending on pharmaceuticals, Switzerland was second behind the United States at $894. Canada spends $879. France spends $671, and Norway $473.[2] A RAND Corporation report on thirty-two countries based on 2018 data concluded that prescription drug prices in the United States are more than two-and-a-half times higher than the other thirty-one countries. While generics account for 84 percent of drugs sold in the United States, they amount to only 12 percent of spending. Brand-name drugs drive the higher drug prices in the United States. Considered apart from generics, these brand-name drugs are nearly three-and-a-half times as expensive as they are in other nations.[3]

Americans are not necessarily taking more medications than people in other countries so much as we are paying more for brand-name drugs, and even some generics, because we have a profit model for our medications. In other countries, governments play a more proactive role in managing costs. Our system leaves a lot of room for people of faith to find creative ways to fill in the gaps because the need is great.

Cure the Sick. The Kingdom Is Near.

The Bible is clear that God's people should care for the poor, the sick, the widows and orphans, the strangers. Old Testament laws provided for people living on the margins of Israel's society. Ruth, for example, was the widow of an Israelite man and an immigrant who cared for her widowed mother-in-law. She made a living gathering grain that harvesters missed because the law of Moses told landowners to leave extra crop for the disadvantaged. Ruth picking up the leftovers that the people of means would never miss seems like an apt image when I think about all the energy over the years to find medications for uninsured patients and how many of those pills came through channels that were originally targeted toward the people who could easily cover the cost at the pharmacy and didn't really need the savings of a box of seven free pills.

Healing is everywhere in the Bible to demonstrate how much God cares. The prophet Elijah raised a widow's only son from the dead. Speaking with the authority God gave him, Elisha told Naaman, a military officer, how to treat his skin disease—and Naaman learned to listen to people outside of his own station in life. Jesus healed people practically every time he turned around—the lame, the blind, the deaf—and expected his followers to do the same. The early church recognized this responsibility and organized itself with a system to care for those in need as well as to offer healing. The good news of God's love doesn't come without the demonstration of God's presence.

Christians in first-century Corinth squabbled—a lot, apparently. They quarreled about allegiance to leaders. They argued about the essence of the gospel message. They debated the pros and cons of participating in the culture around them. Are we so different? They jockeyed to get the "best" gifts for ministry and worship and Christian living. What we know about that one congregation is a compelling argument that nothing much is new in the church. Paul's answer is just as enduring: Remember, above all things, you are the body of Christ. One Spirit baptizes believers into one body.

"You are the body of Christ."

A body is a visible, palpable, physical presence. If we are the body of Christ, shouldn't we be doing what Jesus did?

Christians should be concerned about health care for people who can't afford doctors or medications. Why? The simple answer is, of course, because Jesus was. And we are the body of Christ.

Jesus healed. Sick people came to him in droves, and he exhausted himself with a healing ministry as much as a preaching ministry. The two were intertwined. When Jesus sent the first disciples out in pairs, he said, "Cure the sick who are there, and say to them, 'The kingdom of God has come near to you'" (Luke 10:9). Jesus sent them not only to preach the kingdom of God but also to heal as a demonstration of the kingdom's presence and power. Healing is as much a part of the gospel message today as it was in the first century.

Jesus hasn't changed. But have we? Do we welcome the sick as Jesus did? Do we embrace our work—all of us in the church—to heal just as those pairs did in Luke 10? A lot of people even with insurance grumble about the cost of medications, and there is good reason to think something is wrong with the system. When we look at the issues through the eyes of people who are uninsured and working in low-wage jobs and making choices between putting food on the table and paying for pills that can keep them from having a stroke, that sure fires up our sense of injustice.

Are we hearing Jesus's voice? Am *I* hearing his voice? That's a question I ask myself every day. When you meet people like Bobbie and John and Maxine, I hope you'll ask it too.

For Reflection

1. In your own experience or in connection to a loved one who has needed medication for an illness or to manage chronic disease, what underlying assumptions have you had about the availability and affordability of medications? How are those assumptions similar to or different from the stories in this chapter?

2. Many people talk about the problem of "Big Pharma" in the US healthcare system. Have you ever thought through your own views on how the pharmaceutical industry both helps and hinders health care? Try to summarize them in one or two sentences.

3. In what ways does your personal faith inform your thoughts about justice in relation to the accessibility to affordable medications?

FIVE

BACK TO WORK WITH DUCT-TAPED KNEES AND BROKEN SMILES

Melvin would show up for a bartending job and people would say, "I'm going to get you a chair."

"Man, I don't want to be like that." Melvin "Too Tall" Moore was clearly despondent as he told me of his struggles. "I want to be me again."

I felt the anguish in his voice.

I first met Too Tall almost thirty years ago as I began getting to know people who would contribute to the financial backbone of Church Health. I was invited to private parties, and it seemed that at almost each one, Too Tall was the bartender. A big Black man—six foot five inches tall—with a big heart to match, he makes you feel like he has known you forever even if he's meeting you for the first time. His smile is big. His hands are big. His voice is big, and he is never more than a moment from a big belly laugh. I've always been impressed with the way he treats some of the wealthiest people in Memphis just like he was part of their family.

Early on I would gravitate to him because I felt like a stranger at the parties except to the host, and Too Tall was willing to talk to me about anything.

He grew up in Collierville, Tennessee, which is now an affluent suburb of Memphis. When he was a child, it was very much a rural community. His mother picked cotton before she began working domestic jobs. Too Tall is the middle of five children. These days he is known all over town simply as Too Tall, but he used to ask his mom, "Why am I the only one without a middle name or a nickname?" He was just Melvin.

When he was in the fifth grade, his mom moved the family to north Memphis. His father was never in the picture. "I didn't have a lot of good days growing up," he told me. Because he was from the country, he was picked on in school when they moved to town. "I ran home almost every day." He did this to avoid fights.

When it came time to go to high school, he chose Tech High even though it meant he would have to ride the city bus to get there, and he was always scrounging up bus fare. He graduated in 1977 and went to Tennessee State. Eventually he got a degree in restaurant management, but even with a college education, a young Black man had only two job options: a sacker at Kroger or a busboy at the restaurant Four Flames.

Melvin chose Four Flames, but he didn't know a soup spoon from a salad fork. Nevertheless, he stayed there for ten years, rising to become the maître d'. While he worked there, his sister was teaching school in Memphis City Schools and worked at night as a bartender for the Memphis Country Club. Historically, this is the most exclusive club in Memphis. Only company CEOs and professionals were invited to be members. One night the maître d' of the club's restaurant convinced Melvin to come work for him. He was twenty-three years old and his son, also named Melvin, had just been born. Thus began his long road of working two or three jobs at a time.

He started as a waiter, determined to make a better life for his son. "I didn't have a father figure in my life. I wanted him to grow up knowing better."

When Melvin started working at the country club, Ed "Too Tall" Jones was playing for the Dallas Cowboys. People knew that he had gone to Tennessee State as did Melvin, so since he was also tall they started calling him Too Tall. He didn't like it at first, but he got used to it. He told me, "A lot of people come up to me and ask, 'Too Tall, what's your name?' I tell them, but they keep calling me Too Tall."

A few years ago, Melvin's wife lost her health insurance. Melvin had been on her policy. So when he started to feel numb on his right side, he was afraid he'd had a stroke, but he couldn't afford a doctor. One of the physicians he bartended for ruled out stroke as the cause of his numbness, which was a relief, but the problem didn't go away. By the time he came to see me, he'd been putting up with it for more than two years. He was weak in his right arm and leg, and his sensations were not normal. I arranged for an MRI of his neck. A disc had ruptured and was pressing on the nerve. He needed surgery. One of the best neurosurgeons in Memphis did the operation for free, and everything seemed to be heading in the right direction.

Only the problem came back.

Now Melvin was working three jobs and struggling to keep up. He started drinking heavily to dull the pain. A couple of times when I saw him at parties, he'd clearly had too much to drink. I convinced him to come back and see me.

When I walked into the exam room, he tried to be upbeat, but he could hardly stand up. A small push could have made him fall over.

He sat back down with tears in his eyes. "I need to get myself back to normal."

That was not going to happen any time soon. Or ever.

Maybe in the Winter

Paul is ten years younger than I am, but he looks ten years older. When I first shook his hand, I felt hard callouses, clearly from years of strenuous manual labor—the type of work I had never done.

The only time I worked doing real labor was during the summer after my freshman year in college. I worked on a construction crew in Daytona Beach, Florida, and, with little skill, was assigned to use a shovel to dig footers, the precursor to pouring concrete for a foundation. In the scorching hot Florida sun, it was the hardest thing I have ever done. I quit after two weeks. I knew I wouldn't make it through the whole summer. My friend Ken, who was with me, and I started our own "painting company," even though neither of us had ever painted a thing. It was bound to be a much easier job than holding a shovel eight hours a day while our brains fried in the Florida sun. It was not as easy as we hoped, but it beat the constant intensive challenge of cracking through the earth.

It was not just Paul's hands that were weathered. His face had the lines that come with being outside day after day in all kinds of weather. His hair was short and curling and had turned gray just like mine. He wore a white work shirt with the name of the company he worked for stitched over the left pocket. His shoes were thick, steel-toed boots. His smile was infectious. He was extremely polite, saying "Yes, sir" or "No, sir" to me as I asked him questions about why he came to the doctor.

I had watched him walk into the examining room from the waiting room, and I had already guessed why he was there. He limped on his right leg, and I suspected he had a problem with his right knee.

As soon as we began to talk, I felt drawn to him. I treat many women his age for an array of problems, but I have a much smaller number of Black men as patients. Black men simply don't come to the doctor unless there is something whoa bad wrong.

When I asked Paul, "What can I do for you today?" he didn't go into a long story with details. He just cut to the chase.

"Doc, there's something wrong with my knee. Can you fix it?"

I tried to unravel the problem. "How long has it been bothering you?"

"A while."

I get this answer often. "How long is a while?"

Paul looked up to the ceiling. "Oh, it's been a minute."

I knew I wasn't going to pin him down. "Did you hurt it?" I asked.

He got animated. "I didn't do anything. It just started paining me."

"Does it affect your work?" I was certain that it did.

"That's why I am here." He said it kindly, but the implication was clear. I was an idiot to ask such a question.

"What kind of work do you do?"

He quickly replied, "Concrete."

"How long have you been doing concrete?"

"I don't know, since I could walk." He smiled sheepishly at me.

I hadn't yet examined him, but I already sensed what the problem was. I have treated a number of concrete workers over the years, and they all had knee problems.

The first time I ever saw concrete being poured was back during my two weeks of working construction in Florida. The concrete truck poured the soft, liquid goo into a form that had been built, and then very strong men in knee-high boots jumped in and began smoothing out the mess. It seemed like they were icing a cake, only concrete is not butter. It is made up of rocks in a mix that is quickly gelling. Moving around the mixture requires brute strength and may even be done while on your knees. This is the work Paul had been doing for over forty years.

I wanted to know more about him. "Where did you grow up?"

"In Orange Mound." I knew this to be the first Black community in Memphis. Residents of Orange Mound take great pride in their neighborhood.

"So did you go to Booker T. Washington?" I was certain the answer would be yes because that is the historic high school in Orange Mound.

"Yes, sir," Paul said with a hint of pride.

"Did you start your job after you graduated?"

"No, sir, I started when I was in the ninth grade." My upper-middle-class background had assumed he didn't have to work when he was in high school.

"I married my high school sweetheart," he just offered up. It felt like he and I were connecting. I was more interested in learning about him than turning to examine his knee, but I knew I had to keep moving because other patients were waiting.

He took off his pants and I pulled my rolling stool up close to his knee. Without even touching his knee, I could see he had a big problem. His knee was swollen, and the bones were deformed in a way that happens when the joint deteriorates. I put my hands on his knee and raised and lowered it. I could feel something known as crepitus, a creaking sound and feeling that comes about when bone is rubbing on bone. This was not good.

"What do you think, Doc?"

I didn't want to say what I really thought, so I replied, "I can understand why you are hurting. Let's get an X-ray."

"You're the doctor," he said with a laugh.

Looking at the X-ray hurt me when I saw that the joint was almost totally destroyed from arthritis. I know the feeling because I have four artificial joints myself, and I remember what it's like.

My arthritis came about from what I tend to call "bad luck." It certainly didn't come from doing the type of work Paul did. I made the decision to have my first knee replaced just before the 2002 Winter Olympics in Salt Lake City. The Olympic torch came through Memphis, and I was asked to carry it for a quarter of a mile. I decided that you can't walk carrying the Olympic torch. You have to run. So I consciously decided this would be the last time I ever ran. I injected my knee with lidocaine and a steroid, wrapped it in two braces, and then ran down Poplar Avenue in the heart of Memphis carrying the torch. Running with the torch was an extremely satisfying experience. Two weeks later I had the surgery that removed parts of the bones in my leg and replaced them with metal.

When I looked at Paul's X-ray, I knew he would need the same surgery.

I returned to the room and told him what I saw as simply as I could. "Paul, your knee looks like a car tire when it has lost all of its rubber. You are riding on the rim."

"That bad, Doc? So can you fix me?"

I knew he wanted a pill or a simple fix.

"Paul, when you don't have any more rubber, you usually have to replace the tire." I paused.

"Doc, I got a big job to do. Can you get me fixed up for now?" What Paul had to do was more important than my running with the Olympic Torch, but I hoped I could buy him some time by giving him a steroid injection in his knee.

When injecting a knee, the steroid is mixed with lidocaine, a numbing agent, so after I was done, Paul said, "Doc, you have fixed me. It doesn't hurt. You are a great doctor."

I wanted to think he was right, but I knew it wouldn't last. "Come back if it starts to hurt again," I told him and shook his hand and said goodbye.

Six weeks later he returned. "Doc, can you give me another one of those shots?"

I knew it wouldn't make much difference. I pulled my trouser legs up and showed him the scars on my two knees. "Paul, I have had both of my knees replaced. The time has come that we need to change your tire."

He was quiet. "I see. How much will that cost?"

I then explained to him how we had a surgeon who would do the surgery for free. The hospital wouldn't charge him. Smith and Nephew, the prosthesis manufacturer, would donate the artificial joint. Nor would he get any other big bills. I told him with great pride and enthusiasm that it was a small miracle, but the very expensive surgery would be done almost free for him.

Again he was quiet. I sat on the stool looking up at him, waiting for him to say, "Let's get it done." But those words never came.

After a while I asked, "Is there a problem?"

He looked at me earnestly. "Will I have to miss work?"

My stomach sank. I understood the issue. Paul is the primary breadwinner for his family, and I suspected several other people depended on his tireless work.

But we were going to replace his knee. It was major surgery. After both of my knee replacements, I thought I was going to die at first. Then I suffered through physical therapy for weeks. I made it back into the office and worked at my desk, but it was another month before I started seeing patients again, and I did that with a cane. I had no idea how long it would have taken me to get back to work doing concrete.

"Yes, Paul, you will need to miss six to eight weeks of work, and maybe longer, before you can do what you are used to doing."

He was again very quiet. "I thought so," he said softly. Then after a few more seconds he regained his positive attitude and said enthusiastically, "Maybe after it gets cold this winter we can do that, but I've got lots of work this summer. For now, the duct tape works just fine."

He was not joking. I understood what he meant. He had developed a way every morning of using duct tape to strap his knee in place so that he could make it through the day.

My admiration for him grew.

"I understand," I said as positively as I could. "I tell you what. Let me give you another shot today. Then I am going to have you see our physical therapist to try and give you some ways to manage for now, and we will make a plan that come winter we will do the surgery. How does that sound?" It was the best plan I could come up with.

Once again, after the injection the pain was momentarily gone, and he thanked me for being a great doctor.

I let Kevin, our lead physical-rehabilitation therapist, know Paul would be coming. He was up for the challenge.

As the summer went on, I often thought about Paul, especially if I passed a construction site. He didn't return to the office until just after Thanksgiving.

When I walked in to see him, he was all smiles. "I'm ready."

I could tell he was ready because he was hardly walking. The visit didn't take long. I knew what I needed to do. I put in the order to see the joint-replacement surgeon. Unfortunately, I knew Paul would not be seen until January. Orthopedists are the busiest in December because people have met their health insurance deductibles late in the calendar year and want expensive surgery done before the end of the year and their out-of-pocket costs start all over again. Since the surgeon would be volunteering, we would need to wait until January to replace Paul's knee.

I could see the disappointment on his face. He tried not to show it. "I got you, Doc. I understand. You just let me know, and I'll be here."

It turned out that Dr. Owen Tabor Jr. was willing to see Paul in December to get ready for the surgery in early January. Owen has been volunteering to replace joints for us since his father, Owen Tabor Sr., introduced him to me. His father began volunteering when we first opened in 1987. When Owen Jr. joined his practice, he fell in line in a big way. He never said no, and he worked closely with the hospital and Smith and Nephew to make sure that all the components that can generate a bill were covered.

When it came time for my second joint replacement, I turned to Owen. It was the same for my third and fourth. I knew Paul would get the same care Owen gave me.

I also turned to Owen when one of the biggest donors and supporters of Church Health fell and broke her hip and needed hip-replacement surgery. Weetie Phillips and her husband, Harry, took me on like a sixth son early on, in addition to the five others they already had. After Harry's death, I tried to give back by helping her every way I could. When Weetie fell in her early eighties, it was certain she would need surgery, and the family turned to me to pick the surgeon. I chose Owen because of my experience with him and because I knew that Weetie and Harry had been friends of the Tabor family for many years.

Weetie was a very prim and proper woman whom I loved dearly. She always treated me kindly, so when I told her she would need surgery, she took it in stride. But when I told her Owen would be her surgeon, she was adamant.

"No, he is not doing my surgery. Get someone else."

I was stunned. "Weetie, Owen is a great surgeon. I know he will do a good job."

She was insistent. "He is not doing it."

I kept pushing. I didn't understand. I finally asked point blank, "Weetie, why won't you let Owen do the surgery?"

She was direct. "Because I changed his diapers."

That I didn't expect. We got through it. He did the surgery, and she did fine, and I knew that Paul would have the same outcome.

Paul showed up for his pre-surgery medical clearance. It was an easy exam. He was healthy as a horse. He would do well. I wrote the letter, and the surgery was scheduled. I told him that he would come to us for his physical rehabilitation when he got out of the hospital.

Paul was ready to go but had little understanding of what was about to happen. Many people who work all day long have no reason to be familiar with hospitals and the health-care system. It can be very frightening when the day comes. I was nervous for Paul, but I knew he would not have any major problems.

When the surgery was over, Owen sent me a text. "Mr. Paul did well. Thank you for letting me help care for him." Owen wouldn't get paid a penny. He was thanking me, but I knew he meant it. The experience of caring for Paul made his life better. I was sure of it.

Two weeks later I was walking through our physical rehabilitation clinic. Kevin was in the corner working with a man on his knee. It is what he is often doing, so I didn't pay much attention.

"Hey, Doc," the man on the couch called to me.

It was Paul. I walked over. "So how are you doing?" Looking at him, I knew he was only now getting to the point where he could believe he would walk again. The physical therapy was still very hard.

"When do you think I can get back to work?" That is the most common question I get asked from our working patients. If they don't work, they don't get paid. If they don't get paid, their families don't eat.

"Kevin, how is he doing?" I turned to see what Kevin thought.

"He's doing great. We're making progress." Progress to me and Kevin was probably not what Paul meant. He would get there, but it was still six or eight weeks away.

I replied, "I know it doesn't seem like it, but the pain will be gone soon, and you will get your life back. It won't be what God first gave you, but you'll be back."

He smiled broadly. "I trust you, Doc."

Those words weigh heavy on me. I am not sure that trust in me is what Paul or anyone else should be expressing, but when there is no one else looking out for you, you need to find someone to trust. I accept the responsibility.

"We'll get you back working soon, Paul. Just do what Kevin tells you. Don't make me have to get on you for slacking off. Plus, we are done with the duct tape on your knee. You can use it for something else."

He gave a big laugh. "You're the boss. You can count on me."

Paul's knee will never be how it was twenty years ago, but the pain will be gone and he can do most normal things. I worry about how his artificial knee will take the stress of concrete work. I have never tried to run since I carried the Olympic torch, although many people return to active sports after joint-replacement surgery. I limit my aerobic activity to the elliptical. It is easy on my joints, and I know it gives me the best chance for my joints to last the rest of my life. Paul won't have the luxury of that choice. But I believe we have done the best we could for him, and this gives me peace.

A Dental Minefield

Jorge was a sweet boy with a round face and jet-black hair. He wore a Dallas Cowboys T-shirt, but I don't think he knew much about American football. As I do with most children his age, I asked him and not his mother why he had come to see me. He looked shocked and glanced at his mother.

"I asked you, not her," I said with a smile.

"I have a sore throat." His nasal sound told me his nose was also stopped up. I would have little to offer him for a viral upper respiratory infection.

"What grade are you in?"

He smiled and said, "Third."

"Do you like your teacher?"

"Yes." I could tell he liked my asking him these questions. "Do you have a girlfriend?"

Clearly I caught him off guard.

"No!"

"I don't know. I bet the girls like you," I kidded him.

"They do not!"

I tapped the end of the examining table. "Sit up here and let me take a look at you."

He jumped up on the table and I came close. He smiled at me with pretty, white teeth. "Open your mouth for me."

His mouth was a dental minefield. Multiple teeth had large holes, and several had been filled before only to have the amalgam falling out now. This was not the first time I had seen a child whose mouth looked like this. In fact, over the years it has become a common sight.

The cause is almost always related to the children's diet. It usually begins when they are infants. Because the mother is often working, she does not breastfeed for more than a few weeks. She quickly switches to a bottle. When there are multiple children and limited hands to watch them all, mothers fill bottles, and the children suck on them throughout the day. The constant contact with sugar erodes the enamel of the teeth and creates multiple cavities. Eating other sweets does the same thing when the permanent teeth start coming in. It both creates dental problems at an early age and leads to early obesity. Jorge was also showing signs of being overweight.

I turned to his mom, who was attentively watching everything I did. She was in her early thirties and holding an infant while I examined Jorge.

"His problem today is just a cold. That will get better, but I'm worried about the problems he has with his mouth. He needs to see our dentist."

Listening through Andrea, an interpreter, Jorge's mother agreed for me to set up an appointment for him with the dentist.

Since we have far more medical patients and physicians than we do dentists, it took a few weeks for Jorge to be seen, but I knew our goal would be to restore his mouth. Most physicians have a limited understanding of the importance of dental care. We get patients to open their mouths and say "Ah" pretending the patient does not have teeth. I know for me, in four years of medical school, there was one lecture on teeth, and I fell asleep halfway through it. For the first few years of my practice, I am embarrassed to say, I didn't even know the names of the teeth. I doubt many practicing physicians do.

Jorge's appointment was with Dr. Laurie Hodge, our dental director. Laurie is a young dentist who has taught me the true value of dental care, especially among people facing social and economic challenges. Dental issues affect a person's appearance, which impacts the way the person is perceived in public. This leads to limitations of job opportunities and how a person is regarded in career advancement. Once a front tooth is missing, a person is not put in positions that relate to the public. Others may perceive the person as "dumb." It definitely impacts income over a lifetime.

It also limits one's ability to chew, which leads to eating soft food, which might not be healthy. It is a downward spiral with no good ending. And at age eight, Jorge was well beyond the starting gate for this journey. Laurie was determined not to let it happen with him.

Treating an eight-year-old with extensive dental cavities is no easy task. You must first develop trust. Fixing Jorge's teeth was going to cause some pain. The lidocaine and the drilling are hard for many adults to handle, and it is asking a lot for an eight-year-old to understand the value of what is being done.

Laurie has very long, blond hair that she puts in a bun while she works. These days dentists gown up like they are in the operating room, which in many ways they are. When she puts on her face goggles and paper gown, I suspect she can be scary to a child Jorge's age, but before having him lie down in the chair, she had already won him over.

It was clear she could not fix everything in one day. His treatment plan would take multiple sessions. The first was spent fixing a couple of the worst teeth and ensuring Jorge that she would be gentle with him. After several visits, Laurie had fixed the right side of his mouth, but she still had the left side to go.

She sat him up in the chair and with great enthusiasm told him, "Now we just need to do a few more teeth and we will be finished. Are you ready to get that done?"

To continue to work on a child you have to get his buy-in. No matter how much mom wants it, you can't just force a child to lie down and let you start drilling. The time it takes to do the right work on a child is why many children's dentists who work on the mouths of children in low-income families do such a terrible job.

Medicaid will pay for children to see the dentist but only for limited work. It pays to seal children's teeth, which in theory prevents cavities. However, if the cavities are already present, sealant just makes the problem worse. Because Medicaid pays only a limited reimbursement, dentists all too often use chrome fillings. These silver-colored teeth coverings temporarily stop cavities from developing further, but they are a long way from restoring the dental health of the child. Medicaid reimburses for them because they are quick and cheap.

In Jorge's case, since he was undocumented, even that option was not available to him. Because of Church Health's commitment to quality care, Laurie had the resources to do the right thing for Jorge. We charge on a sliding scale according to the family's income. Jorge's mother would never be able to afford the true cost of the work Laurie was doing, but her portion was around $100 for every visit.

As Laurie was preparing Jorge for the last run that would give him a chance for a healthy mouth as he got older, Jorge had other plans. Laurie asked, "Are you ready for me to finish your mouth?" She said this with great enthusiasm and a smile.

Jorge sat and thought for a minute and then replied, "I think we should wait a little while to do this. My mom needs to work more so that we can pay for this." He said it very matter-of-factly and with the maturity of an older man. He was saying something no eight-year-old should be worried about.

Laurie was speechless. She was talking to Jorge about the return visit because she needed him to buy into the plan and be willing to go through another round of dental procedures and because he was the person in the family who spoke English. But she knew that what he said was wrong in so many ways.

She nodded her head to register that she understood. She didn't want to push the matter, so she got out of her gown and went to tell his mother how he did and that she should make the next appointments when she was ready. She didn't tell her what Jorge had said. I suspect she would have been embarrassed to know.

Prophetess on the Doorstep

The doorbell rang. It was Thanksgiving 2018 in San Jose, California, the heart of Silicon Valley. Angie Bymaster opened the door to her Honduran friend, Ruth, who was a missionary to the United States and went house to house offering prayer.

A prophetess.

Ruth had a prophetic word for Angie, who was struck by the irony. Angie was a young Christian doctor working with the underserved but had become frustrated with the difficulty of caring for the spiritual dimension in people's lives while practicing medicine in a government-funded clinic. Ruth, coming from a poor Central American country, said, "God wants you to start a clinic for the poor." Angie was taken aback. What was she to do with such a pronouncement on her life?

Angie and her minister husband, Brett, had moved to San Jose devoted to the John Perkins model of Christian social action. They moved into the community they sought to care for, became a part of the neighborhood, and joined a multiracial church with strong community outreach. When the Bymasters adopted two South Sudanese sons, their Black children were the only non-Latinx kids in the local school. As a medical resident and beyond, Angie worked in a clinic serving a homeless population, and then for five years she worked in a federally qualified health center (FQHC) in their neighborhood, which allowed her to walk to work.

But it wasn't enough.

Maria was a young patient who came to her with suicidal thoughts. Angie knew Maria from the church where Brett was a pastor and from living in the neighborhood. Domestic violence was a large part of the problem, and Angie believed Maria was experiencing a spiritual void. In the federally funded clinic, Angie felt stymied in caring for the spiritual needs of patients like Maria.

Even Angie's patients with hypertension and diabetes could be better served if there was a way to provide them with the community they lacked. Angie believed that leading those whom she cared for in a way that offered communal nurturing was far better than just writing more prescriptions for pharmaceuticals. She was looking for another path for her career when Ruth knocked at the door.

Throughout the holidays that year, Angie and Brett kept coming back to what Ruth said. "God wants you to start a clinic for the poor." A few weeks later, in January 2019, they Googled "How to start a Christian health clinic." The first thing that popped up was ECHO—Empowering Church Health Outreach—a ministry of Church Health helping to establish faith-based clinics.

They quickly made plans to come to Memphis for a Church Health replication seminar. When they did, they realized they weren't alone in this venture. It wasn't crazy. Or if it was, they weren't the only crazy ones.

Soon after this, Brett went on sabbatical from the church for a few months and took it upon himself to read the entire Bible, cover to cover, in eleven weeks. While reading, he kept working to become clearer about what God was saying to them if they were to start a Christian health clinic based on the work of Jesus. When he got to the New Testament, he asked the question, What was the work of Jesus? That Jesus was a healer was undeniable, but Jesus did not heal just for the sake of healing. As Brett saw it, every time Jesus healed someone, he did so to restore dignity to that person.

He also noted that Jesus healed not only the poor. He healed the centurion's servant and others who were not financially poor. This realization led the Bymasters to a hybrid model of care—concierge medicine for both the well-to-do and those with low incomes.

They live in a predominantly Latinx community, so one-third of the patients speak Spanish, and most are undocumented. At the same time, the Bymasters are in Silicon Valley in the heart of the world of social media and the internet, so another one-third of the people who might be patients in a concierge practice work for Google or Apple, and another one-third are others who are able to afford a concierge doctor. Those who can afford the cost of concierge medicine—drawing heavily from the church to start with and expanding to other congregations—will also be underwriting the cost of quality care for the underserved in the community.

Healing Grove Health Center was incorporated in January 2020. They began work to restore a space for the clinic. Grants and financial support came pouring in. On March 12, as planned, Angie quit her job at the FQHC to become full-time at the Healing Grove clinic. On February 6, 2020, the first COVID-19 death in the United States occurred in San Jose. The timing could not have been worse.

But God had called them to this work, and they were ready. The FQHC clinic Angie had worked for was not prepared to do COVID-19 testing, and in fact it shut down. Angie and Brett began doing COVID-19 testing in the parking lot before they even had their clinic space up and going. Since they had lived in this community for fifteen years by this time, people trusted them, and they knew how important their neighbors were to the economy of the city. Their neighbors, now patients, were responsible for everything that seemed to matter. They built everything. They grew the food, they harvested the food, they cooked it, and they cleaned up. They cared for children; they worked in nursing homes. They were essential but did not receive dignity or honor. The very dignity that Brett saw Jesus restoring when he reached out to heal was often missing in their work and certainly in the time of COVID-19.

The Bymasters had found their calling.

Throughout 2020, challenges continued to present themselves as they expanded the common understanding of health. Barriers sprouted up everywhere. Because they knew the local networks and resources, the Bymasters worked with community leaders to find ways to distribute food to the community and keep rents paid. No one received stimulus relief dollars or unemployment benefits because everyone was undocumented, so the Bymasters called on their church to be what they understood church to be and got rolling. Issues of housing, childcare, food, and clothing were all part of what this new health clinic took on. Maria has become a patient in the new clinic. Her issues are still present, but she is learning to trust Angie in new ways. The road is still long, but building up trust is making a difference, and now Angie has the freedom to address the whole of Maria's life by not being limited to treating only her clinical issues.

When people got sick, they were reluctant to go to the federally funded clinic because they knew it was hard for people who were undocumented to know who to trust when there are government connections to services. Angie and Brett let it be known that the church is open to all. After working on rehabbing their space during the early months of the COVID-19 crisis while also scrambling to alleviate the virus-induced poverty in the neighborhood, the concierge clinic opened its doors in June 2020.

The concierge practice was slow to take off at first, but employees of Google and Apple seem to like knowing that their $200 a month helps two other people who are uninsured to receive care. This covers unlimited primary care, physician access, help navigating the health-care system, and invitation to programs that care for the whole person. Healing Grove also has minimal cost rates that cover entire low-income families and reduced-fee plans to help remove barriers to care. They are working toward a model of one-third concierge care and two-thirds care for uninsured and low-income patients. Along with donations, the model is moving in the right direction.

Angie and Brett's energy for the work is palpable. They have found their sense of purpose.

In the early fall of 2020, Prophetess Ruth returned from Honduras and rang Angie and Brett's doorbell. Her word from God this time was, "Just care for my people and I will pay for it."

In Seattle, Washington, another concierge practice focused on pediatrics is also leveraging this model to give people with low incomes the same access to this high level of care that people with more substantial incomes gain by subscribing to the practice. The Hope Central Health

Clinic also integrates behavioral health and clinical psychologists into its pediatric practice, something that is a big draw to families concerned that their kids might need extra services that most pediatric services don't offer. While serving low-income families, subscribing higher-income families to the practice means a financial model not entirely dependent on charity. However, education helps supporters from churches and elsewhere understand the transformative value of their gifts in the lives of the patients who benefit.

I have been told for over thirty years that the Church Health model isn't sustainable. I completely understand this sentiment. Anything that depends on the kindness and generosity of others easily looks like foolishness. Health care in the United States is one-sixth of our national economy, so most people believe that a transactional business plan is the only way to provide health care. I am not arguing that a faith-based model is a better business model for health care. However, I do believe that being faithful to what God has called us to do in this world requires us to engage in a healing ministry. What form this takes can vary. The Bymasters in San Jose and the team at Hope Central in Seattle work in a manner very different from our work in Memphis, Tennessee. For all of us, though, I hope that our efforts reflect what we know of our own communities and help break down the barriers that keep our neighbors from receiving the quality of care they deserve.

God is pushing us forward in a way that brings us closer to God and serves others in ways that affirms the dignity God created in them. That is the reason to do this work.

The Story in Numbers

Lack of health insurance combined with living in poverty leads to poor health outcomes. According to the Kaiser Family Foundation's research, delaying health care for both preventive services and chronic disease leads to worse health outcome in various ways. Using 2019 numbers not skewed by the pandemic (when increasing numbers of people delayed care out of caution against infection), more than one-third of the uninsured have no regular primary care provider, compared to only 7 percent of those with insurance. One in ten adults reported delaying or not receiving care because of the cost. Latinx and Black populations had higher rates of going without care. One in four adults went without dental care, and 12 percent went without prescription drugs because of the expense.[1]

The Affordable Care Act created market-based, subsidized insurance policies, but deductible rates vary. Plans that keep premiums down by using a high deductible often require people to pay the first $5,000 before the policy kicks in. This contributes to even people with insurance delaying care. A 2019 survey of physicians at the University of Chicago found that they believed the high-deductible plans and anxiety about medical debt were a major factor in people's avoiding care.[2] Hospitals often charge uninsured patients higher amounts for services than what they bill for the same services to private health insurance policies or public programs that have negotiated rates. When uninsured individuals are unable to pay the costs—even for one visit to the emergency department, let alone an admission to the hospital—the bills strain financial well-being that is already fragile. Bills end up in collections or even court.[3]

Poverty and a low-income status are associated with shorter life expectancy, higher infant mortality rates, and higher death rates for the fourteen leading causes of death. At the same time, poverty is an obstacle to the resources necessary to adopt healthy behavior and avoid these risks. Where people live, work, and play—buildings, open spaces (if there are any), and infrastructure all bear on health. Location matters dramatically. The Robert Wood Johnson Foundation looked at an inner-city neighborhood and a suburban neighborhood in New Orleans and found a twenty-five-year difference in life expectancy even though the two neighborhoods were only a few miles apart. Two neighborhoods in Kansas City, Missouri, that are three miles apart had a difference in life expectancy of fourteen years.[4]

Where people are born, where they grow up, where they work, where they age, their education, how they earn a living, whether they have supportive social networks, whether there are faith communities in the neighborhood, how far it is to a doctor or hospital or a pharmacy, whether stores in the neighborhood carry fresh food or only processed food, whether the bus or train lines are nearby, whether rental housing is maintained in safe conditions and is affordable—these are "social determinants of health."

They are not conditions individuals can solve on their own but rather challenges that call us to work together to close the inequities that result in health care and health outcomes.

Healings from Acts

Peter and Paul, the towering leaders of the early church, preached and taught, but they also healed. Luke recounts nineteen different healing stories in Acts, and likely these were only the highlights. Luke points out more than once that the apostles performed "many wonders and signs" among the people (Acts 2:43; 5:12; 14:3; 19:11). Both Peter and Paul healed people who had never been able to walk. Paul himself received a healing miracle. When he encountered Christ for the first time on the road to Damascus, the experience left him blind. God sent a Christian named Ananias to find Paul and heal him. God demonstrated healing through Paul's ministry so consistently that people brought handkerchiefs and aprons for him to touch and took them back to cure their sick loved ones (Acts 19:12). Even as a Roman prisoner shipwrecked after a bad storm because someone made a stubborn sailing decision, Paul had a healing ministry for strangers on an island (Acts 28:8–9).

Peter and Paul even have resurrection stories. When a woman named Tabitha died while Peter was staying in a nearby town, the Christians went to fetch him. Clearly these believers expected healing was possible even in the face of death. They did not merely report Tabitha's demise. They said, "Please come to us without delay" (Acts 9:38). Peter didn't shrug them off and say there was nothing he could do now that Tabitha was dead. He went with them to see what healing God might choose to do. When Peter arrived to find a mass of mourners crying and remembering Tabitha's life, he did not merely say, "She lived a good life." He dedicated himself to the task of bringing healing. He went upstairs to the room where Tabitha died and where her body still lay, and there he got down on his knees and prayed. Then he said, "Tabitha, get up." And she opened her eyes, saw Peter, and sat up. Peter escorted her back downstairs, a walking and talking announcement of the kingdom of God.

Paul knew a captive audience when he saw one. One Sunday in Troas, the Christians gathered to worship, and Paul was the featured speaker.

Since he planned to leave the next day, he couldn't say, "We'll pick this up next week." Instead, he talked all day and all the way to midnight. A young man named Eutychus sat in an open third-story window. As much as he might have thought he wanted to hear Paul teach, Eutychus got tired and dropped into a sound sleep—and then plummeted to the ground from that third-story window. No doubt Paul lost some of his audience as they rushed to see what happened. In fact, Paul himself went downstairs. Not surprisingly, Eutychus was dead. But Paul threw himself on him and said, "Don't be alarmed, for his life is in him" (Acts 20:10). And it was.

Not every Christian will go around performing miracles and raising the dead; that's up to God, but Jesus calls all who follow him to demonstrate the same priority of healing the whole person, body and spirit, that he showed. He asks us to care about what he cared about—wellness and wholeness. Healing that flows from personal care, preventive activities, medical methods, and technology announces that the kingdom of God is here. We cannot separate healing from the gospel message. If we're going to do what Jesus did and as his first-century followers did, we must find some way to be involved in a ministry of healing. The church—the body of Christ—must show the here-and-now nature of the kingdom of God through healing.

For Reflection

1. Have you ever met anyone like Melvin, Paul, or Jorge, whose socioeconomic circumstances created barriers to receiving needed health-care services? Barriers can include lack of insurance, not being able to afford time off to heal, dental care not being covered, parents working multiple jobs so it's hard to find time for care during business hours, lack of doctors in a neighborhood, and unavailable public transportation. Based on someone you've known personally or just based on reading about the people in this chapter, what perspective do these stories give you personally about how people of faith can respond to these challenges?

2. Have you ever personally been part of a congregational effort to address a health-care injustice? For instance, this might have been in your own community or on a mission trip to another community or even another country. What was the experience like for you? If you haven't had this experience, what might draw you toward it in the future?

3.   The stories from the book of Acts featured in this chapter highlight ac-
      tive healing ministry by the most familiar leaders in the early church
      and even the expectation of other believers that healing would occur.
      How would you express in your own words the way this translates into
      a calling to healing ministry now?

SIX

NO PAPERS, NO HEALTH CARE

I recognized Maria as soon as I walked into the exam room. She is barely five feet tall. Her face is rounder than those of our patients who come from Mexico in a way I have recognized as being from Central America, and her hair is jet-black and long. She wears it pulled back. Her broad smile flashed as soon as she saw me.

I first met her when she brought her children to our walk-in clinic two years earlier. It was November, and she needed to have her children immunized in order for them to go to school. They had just arrived in Memphis, and even though her children had been immunized before they left Honduras, she did not have the paperwork, so they had to start all over again. The six-year-old, Jesús, winced a bit as he received five shots, but he refused to let himself cry. His seven-year-old sister, Juanita, cried briefly and then pulled close to her mom's side. Maria was just happy we made it as easy as possible for her as we walked her through what she needed to do for the children to begin school.

Since that day, I have treated Maria because of irregular periods. At first she bled heavily for two months straight and didn't come to the doctor because she was afraid both of the cost and that seeking help might lead to her being deported. Through it all, she kept cleaning five houses every week.

She finally screwed up her courage and came to Church Health through our walk-in clinic, where she saw me again. I could tell she was relieved it was me but also afraid. When I told her I would need to order an ultrasound, she balked.

I said, "It won't hurt. They will just spread a little grease on your stomach."

She shook her head. That was not her concern. I immediately knew the problem.

I did my best to comfort her. "Don't worry. You will not get a big bill, and you will not need to miss but a couple of hours of work."

Hearing this, she agreed to go for the test.

Thankfully, I was able to solve the problem with medicine. She was back on track. Through all this, though, I realized that neither Maria nor her children had ever been to the dentist. All the family's teeth were in bad shape. I assumed her husband's teeth were the same, but I have never met him because he is always working. But Maria, now that she trusted me, took the children to our dental clinic, and after coaxing, agreed to go herself.

Now, on this day, Maria was in the room with someone else I had never met. Her name was Wendy, and she was not doing very well.

Like Maria, Wendy was small in stature and had the look of being of native Central American ancestry. It seemed like she must have worked outside. Her hands had thick calluses, and her teeth were in even worse shape than Maria's had been. She was struggling to sit up straight in the chair.

I listened to her heart, which was beating fast. Her mouth was dry, her eyes sunken, her skin doughy. It was the middle of August in Memphis, during which time it is not unusual to see patients with the symptoms of dehydration, but Wendy was on the verge of being seriously depleted.

I turned to Maria and asked her to tell me the story. Because of my past relationship and the trust we'd established, she began the account without hesitation.

Desperate on the Border

Wendy was Maria's cousin and was living in a rural village on the Honduras-Guatemala border. Her husband had been killed by a gang and she had been abused. Worried for her children, she was desperate and reached out to Maria with the hope that she could help her come to the United States. Wendy sold everything she had and, with her two small children, began walking across Mexico headed to the United States.

They were able to take a couple of buses and slept on the side of the road. When she got close to the Texas border, Wendy met other sojourners who introduced her to a "coyote" who promised Wendy he could get her across the border if she paid him $10,000. She didn't have anywhere near that much money!

At first he walked away from her, but after a couple of days he came back. He seemed like a nice man. He was kind to her children. He agreed to take her for all the money she had, about $1,500.

They got up to the border at night. There were about ten others in the group Wendy was with. The coyote left to go scout out their crossing plan and never came back. So near to her goal but with no money and no way to cross, Wendy felt broken. She *was* broken—alone with no plan B.

She managed to call Maria, who didn't hesitate. She arranged for a friend to help her husband watch their children, and she headed to the Texas border. Apparently, if you want to cross the border headed toward Mexico, no one tries to stop you. Maria walked into Mexico without difficulty and wound her way to the place where Wendy was waiting.

Maria was single-minded. She only spent one night and then gathered up the children with Wendy and headed toward the desert and the US border.

It was a frightening journey, terribly hot during the day and cold at night. They were constantly watching for other coyotes who might be looking to rob them or even worse.

They were running low on water when by fate, or providence, they happened on water jugs that Americans had left in the desert for people just like them. Wendy made sure her children had enough to drink but did not drink enough herself. After three days they made it to a town where they could catch a bus to Memphis.

They had just gotten to Maria's home the previous night when Maria realized Wendy was sick and brought her to the walk-in clinic.

After fully examining her, I was comfortable that Wendy would soon recover from her severe dehydration. But as I moved around the examining room, I noticed Maria was limping.

I asked her, "Are you all right?"

She brushed me off. "I'm okay."

"No, you're not. Let me look at your ankle." I made her sit on the examining table and take her shoe off. Her right ankle was swollen and tender. It was also blue. When I went to move it, she winced. "I need to take an X-ray."

She didn't stop me.

"How did this happen?" I asked.

She went on to tell me how she had stumbled at night in the desert.

The X-ray showed that she had broken the part of her ankle formed by the fibula. She had fractured her ankle and then walked on it for two days. Thankfully, it would not need surgery.

I told her, "Maria, I need to put a cast on your foot. You will need to wear it for six weeks, and you need to not put any weight on it for two weeks."

She shook her head. "I can't do that. My husband has lost his job, and I am the only one who is working. Now there are three more mouths to feed."

My stomach sank. This kind woman had risked her own safety in Memphis to help her traumatized cousin cross a desert at night under terrible circumstances, and in doing so she had broken her ankle and would now be at risk of having no income at this critical time. How could this be? I didn't know what to do. I knew I had to put the cast on and tell her what I thought was needed for the bone to heal right. What else could I do unless I was prepared to take them all into my home? And I wasn't ready to do that.

"God has cared for us so far," Maria said. "I am sure he will not abandon us now." A calm seemed to settle over her as she accepted what she needed to do.

Over the next few weeks, I saw both Wendy and Maria back in the office. Wendy quickly recovered as I hoped she would. After two weeks I was able to put Maria into a walking cast so she could work. Wendy's children enrolled in school. They received immunizations in our clinic, and it was as though this was how it had always been, safe for now after what they'd been through.

Maria and Wendy both risked everything to keep people they loved safe and to experience again the simple, normal joys of life. In God's eyes, our obligation is to treat each other—all people—with the dignity we have because we are created and loved by God. It cannot be that in our clinic we would ever turn away from Maria and Wendy and their children because they don't have the same paperwork we do.

The Story in Numbers

One day in the clinic, my first ten patients spoke ten different languages: Spanish, Chinese, Hindi, Russian, Portuguese, French, Creole, an indigenous dialect from Guatemala, Sudanese, and Arabic. This was in Memphis, not New York City. The immigrant population in the United States is on the rise, and it isn't just about the southern border. In 2019 there were 44.93 million foreign-born immigrants in the United States. Only 11.39 million were unauthorized.[1]

In our clinics, we employ five Spanish-speaking interpreters who help with our most frequent language issue for immigrants from Mexico and Central America, but our experience shows that immigration isn't just about people crossing the border illegally. Of 11.39 million unauthorized immigrants in 2019, 47 percent were Mexican, but this was the first time that the Mexican portion had fallen below 50 percent.[2]

Since our clinic depends on donated services and finding ways to help people who are uninsured, it is important for me to understand a patient's immigration status. Some of our methods of getting things done are not available to someone who is uninsured. For instance, if someone needs a kidney transplant but has no insurance and no ability to pay for the expensive antirejection drugs needed for a lifetime, the transplant surgeons understandably can't do the surgery. The surgery might be a success, but the patient will die because the body will reject the transplanted kidney without the antirejection medications.

I try to be matter-of-fact when asking the question through an interpreter, but I know the answer almost immediately when I ask about immigration status. The person's shoulders slump. There is silence. The patient pauses, not understanding why I need to know, but almost always the response is honest. When someone says, "I am illegal," I always correct them and say, "You are unauthorized or undocumented." When I do that, I win the patient over to knowing I am an advocate. No one should ever have to feel defined as an "illegal," especially people who have been working for years in our community, paying taxes and being our neighbors.

Despite the attention on the southern border, most unauthorized immigrants today arrive on a legal visa and then overstay their visa's approval. Ninety percent of unauthorized immigrants are from somewhere other than Mexico and Central America.[3]

Many patients we see are seeking asylum based on fears from their home country. However, their chances of being granted asylum are very small. Only 46,508 people were granted asylum in 2019.[4]

Surprising to many, most unauthorized immigrants have lived in the United States for over fifteen years. Only 20 percent have been in the country for fewer than five years.[5] Unauthorized immigrants constitute 4.6 percent of the US labor force.[6]

No matter who is in the White House, the news cycle never seems to stop debating immigration policy or what to do about the millions of undocumented immigrants who have been living in the United States, perhaps for decades. What is our response as people of faith who believe each person is created by God in God's image? How does our response help all persons, regardless of immigration status, experience the level of health and health care that will help them know the fullness of life God intends for all of us?

Who Are the Called?

Immigrants who cross the border the way Maria and Wendy did, coming from horrific circumstances in search of safety and stability, are not the only people who might lack the documents that give them access to the traditional US health-care system. Individuals or families who are chronically housing insecure—homeless—are another category that can find it hard to navigate the system.

You need an address to apply for identification documents, and the address needs to be current to receive the mailed documents—like a driver's license or state ID card or a replacement social security card, if you can come up with enough proof of identity to get these items issued to you. Finding employment, cashing a check, receiving food stamps or disability benefits, and in some instances getting a bed at a shelter depend on ID. So can going to the doctor, even if logically you should qualify for Medicaid or Medicare.

Just as people find themselves without permanent homes for all sorts of reasons, they can find themselves without necessary proof of identity for all sorts of reasons, making it difficult to re-establish secure employment and housing even when they want to.

One of the people I've admired most in my life has devoted her own life to living among those who have no homes and doctoring some of the most marginalized citizens in our society.

When I was a young doctor, Janelle Goetcheus sat on an old, worn couch in my office while I sat in a wooden chair directly opposite her. I was so thankful she had come to Memphis to speak to our supporters about the work we were both committed to around faith and health for the under-served. It was the summer of 1988. She was the person who, in 1978, had convinced me that starting a faith-based health clinic was doable. From the first time we met, I hung on her every word. I considered her to be a living saint, an attribute I am sure she would deny. By 1988, Janelle had founded, or helped to found, multiple programs that addressed issues impacting the health of very low-income and housing-insecure populations in Washington, DC.

As was always the case, she spoke in a very soft voice but with passion for the cause. Despite her own personal commitment, you could feel the burden of the mission she seemed to carry. Her hair had not changed since I first met her. It was now getting gray, but it was cut in her signature page boy style. She looked like a nun, even though I knew she was married to a Methodist minister and had three children. Around her neck hung a cross that she had worn every time I ever saw her. As she sat on the couch, I peppered her with question after question. Should we do this? Should we do that?

She patiently answered them all. And then when there was a pause in the air, she looked at me tenderly and said forcefully, "You will need to stop calling me!"

I sat back in my chair. I didn't know what to think. I swallowed hard and said, "Come again?"

"Everything you are asking of me needs to come from the 'called people.'"

I shook my head. "Who are the called people?"

"You know who they are. They are the people like yourself, who have come to be a part of this ministry because God has called them here for this purpose."

I nodded. "Yes." I almost instantaneously knew what she meant. She was referring to Kim Simmons, the first employee I ever hired who worked at the front desk. Now, thirty-five years later, she is still with me and has had a dozen different positions over the years, but her sense of calling has never wavered. She has gotten married, had a baby, sent her baby to college, cared for her father when he had a stroke, and watched hundreds of people come and go working near her. Through it all Kim's commitment to the work has remained constant. She knew she was called and still does. Janelle was talking about Ann Langston, who was the sharp attorney at my side in front of the city council when we were trying to open and who later came on staff and only recently retired. She meant so many others who have signed on at Church Health over the years because of the strength of our mission and have had the staying power to grow in their gifts along with us because they were called.

Since that time, I have only seen Janelle a handful of times, although I think of her often. Her work in Washington, DC, is legendary among people who care about faith and health and health care for the underserved. She is often referred to by Washington, DC, politicians as "the Mother Teresa of Washington health care," a term she tries to interrupt as soon as it begins to come out of someone's mouth. But it's true.

Janelle grew up in Indiana, where she went to medical school. In 1976 she and her husband, Al, were headed overseas to be medical missionaries. While waiting for their visas, they spent time in Washington, DC, where they met Gordon Cosby, the founder and pastor of the Church of the Saviour. Gordon's view of ministry was to take very seriously the call to care for the marginalized. You couldn't join the church without first dedicating yourself to an hour of prayer a day and then being fully engaged in one of the church's many ministries focused on serving those in need. Many distinctive ministries grew out of small groups of people discerning a call to address a specific need. While visiting, Janelle saw the need for health care in the shadow of the nation's capital. Gordon showed Janelle and Al the need, and God spoke to them on the spot. Instead of going overseas, they moved to Washington, DC, and joined the Church of the Saviour. A mission group committed to start a clinic. And so was born Columbia Road Community Health Center in 1976.

Bound to Jesus

In 1978, I was in Chicago and learned of a conference organized by Christian Community Health Fellowship. It was a new organization to me, still a seminary student. On a lark, I decided to attend. Janelle was the keynote speaker. I was hooked.

When she was finished speaking, I asked if I could visit her in Washington. She graciously invited me. A few months later, I found my way to DC.

The clinic was small and in an old storefront. I had an appointment with Janelle. When I got there, the front desk receptionist didn't have me on the calendar. Also, Janelle wasn't even there. She was at a clinic for the homeless at a soup kitchen called SOME, So Others May Eat. This was another of the church's ministries that Janelle helped to found. I was told I could go over there and maybe I would find her. I got back in my car and headed out.

When I arrived, the place was overrun with people looking for food. I asked about Dr. Goetcheus. No one seemed to know where she was, so I wandered around, and in the back I found two rooms that had been carved into exam rooms. Janelle was there, acting as receptionist, nurse, and doctor. Her hair was still black then but in the haircut I would come to expect whenever I saw her. The cross hung around her neck. When she greeted me, I was sure she had forgotten I was coming, but she was warm and gracious. While I was still trying to discern my mission in life, I wasn't quite sure why I was there that day. I wasn't a physician yet; I was still a seminary student soon headed to medical school. I felt lost.

Almost immediately, Janelle led us to talk about the call to follow Jesus. Healing the sick, caring for the poor. There was no way to avoid seeing that those two things were what the Gospels expected of Jesus's followers. Janelle was clear; she was in this to be connected to Jesus. "I want to be bound to him," she said. I could feel it with every word she spoke, and I began to better understand what I was supposed to be learning that day.

Several years later, in 1985, I was about to begin my last year of residency, and I went for a Janelle fix. She had undertaken yet another audacious call with a mission group. The Church of the Saviour had just purchased a building and opened what is called Christ House the year before. It is a thirty-three-bed medical recovery shelter for homeless men who are sick and sometimes dying. Hospitals could discharge patients without homes and support Christ House rather than send them back to the grates they were sleeping on that may have led to their becoming sick in the first place, and they would receive care while they recovered. Janelle had seen that uninsured patients were discharged earlier than insured patients, and without some basic care—a bed to rest in, clean surroundings, nutritious food, someone to help change dressings—of course their health outcomes were poor. Christ House became a place where men could not only recover medically but also move to transitional housing and find a turning point in their lives.

The remarkable part of it, for me, was that Janelle and Al had decided that they, with their three young children, would live in Christ House along with the men they were caring for.

It was not an easy decision to make. She worried about what it would mean for her children's education and safety in the neighborhood. Two of them were mugged. She may have felt called to this ministry, but it didn't mean that her children felt the same call. It was anxiety producing and hard on her as a mother, but still they stayed. Today, her children consider Christ House as the best possible place they could have grown up, but at first that wasn't so clear.

When I came for a visit, Janelle arranged for me to stay in a guest room in the dorm. It was a simple room with bunk beds. The shower was down the hall. It was clean, but I questioned in myself if I had the same sense of calling that Janelle had for this ministry. I was a Methodist minister and a doctor. I was willing to dedicate my life to working with the disenfranchised, but I was pretty sure I wasn't ready to live with the homeless in the next room and across the breakfast table. Did that make my calling less valid? I wasn't sure.

Janelle and her family have lived at Christ House since 1985. It is her home. Thousands of men have come and gone. Many of the men have had serious mental illnesses. Others have had substance abuse issues. Christ House takes a holistic approach to support patients in a community setting and help people on the path toward stability. This includes, when necessary, helping men establish their legal identities by finding ways to prove who they are by reconnecting them with family members and navigating systems to get the documents required to access social-safety-net services that can keep them off the streets and give them a way to receive more consistent care in the future. Part of their work has grown to include hospice care. Many men have died while staying at Christ House, but they died knowing they were cared for. Janelle tells the story of a man who got up one morning and came looking for her to speak to her. He then went down for breakfast. He took a shower, he lay down to rest, and he never got up. He died that afternoon. Janelle felt his loss like a member of her family. Later they opened Kairos House to offer longer-term supportive housing for men with chronic illness or who suffer from chronic addiction and are ready for help in recovery.

Because of the experiences of Christ House, Janelle led the charge for the Church of the Saviour to become the primary health-care provider for the homeless and the poor in Washington, DC. From 1995 until she retired, Janelle was the medical director of Unity Health Care, the largest network of community health centers in Washington, DC, for the underserved, including their strong focus on services for people without homes. They serve over a hundred thousand people, with five hundred thousand visits a year in dozens of offices around the city. In 2006 they moved into the Department of Corrections to provide comprehensive medical services in jail facilities with continuing care for patients after they are released.

"These are the things Jesus expects us to do. This is where we find Jesus." It is as simple as that in Janelle's view.

"I was hungry and you gave me food," we hear in Jesus's words about the Son of Man coming in glory. "I was a stranger and you welcomed me, I was naked and you gave me clothing, I was sick and you took care of me, I was in prison and you visited me" (Matthew 25:35–36). And when the righteous say, to paraphrase the following verses, "When? We didn't see you," the king points to "the least of these" and says, "There I was."

We all read this passage. Janelle lives it, along with others in her church community who are formed daily by seeing Jesus in others in their network of healing ministries and experiencing life in community.

Janelle retired in 2019. She now has the title of "emeritus," but she still lives at Christ House. She is still called. She is still looking for Jesus.

I know that my sense of calling is not the same as Janelle's, and yours is bound to be different as well. She doesn't expect us to follow her; she would instead charge us to follow Jesus. "Come, follow me," Jesus said to the first disciples. All he promised was to make them fishers of people, to teach them to be people who would also show others the way to God. Beyond that, they weren't working off a master plan when they left their nets and boats and tax-collector booths and other occupations. As they listened to Jesus preach and teach and watched him heal, they also experienced God in ways they hadn't imagined before.

What does it mean for us to feel called by God to do this work seeing the dignity of people and creating justice in health care? Caring for the underserved and being engaged in health ministry is something we can't ignore if we read the Gospels, but how it looks in our lives can be very different based on what our callings are. Long ago, I found peace in not being Janelle. I just need to keep finding what it means to be Scott, and you will need to do the same in finding what it means to be you in answering God's call.

For Reflection

1. What personal experience do you have with someone who has come into the United States without documentation? Has knowing someone personally influenced your views on "welcoming the stranger"?

2. People may be undocumented because of immigration or because of homelessness—and homelessness may happen for various reasons. How do you feel about the dependence on documents to receive basic health services in our current system?

3. Janelle Goetcheus is an example of someone who has helped many people and inspired many people. Can you think of others about whom this is true in the area of health care?

SEVEN

TACKLING PREVENTABLE CHRONIC DISEASE

"Why do you have to be such an asshole?"

Roger was visibly angry with me and ready to get up to leave. Forty-five years old, he worked long hours repairing cars and had very poor control of his diabetes.

I looked him squarely in the eyes and said, "Because I don't want to be the doctor they call from the emergency room to tell that you have had a stroke. I want you to live a long life and watch your grandkids grow up."

There was a pause. He looked back at me intently and said, "No doctor has ever talked to me before like they cared what happens to me. So what do I need to do?"

Roger was diagnosed with diabetes eight years earlier. He was first given pills, and then about a year ago, he was started on insulin shots. He only took the insulin when he felt bad, though, and as a result his numbers weren't good, especially his hemoglobin A1c. This is a test of the average amount of sugar in a person's blood over a three-month period. Normal for the number is between 4 and 6. As long as the number is below 7, things are okay. It should never go above 9. Every time we tested Roger, he was over 10. It was almost certain something bad was going to happen. I had just told Roger, "If you don't control your blood sugar better, you are going to have a stroke, have a heart attack, go blind, or kill your kidneys, and we will have to cut your legs off. And I want to be perfectly clear. If we cut your legs off, you will not grow new ones."

That's when he, understandably, called me an asshole.

What became clear, as is all too often the case, is that Roger didn't really understand what diabetes is. Once he came to see that I actually had his

best interest at heart, we were ready to start over from square one, beginning with my simpleminded way of explaining diabetes. It wasn't exactly
accurate, but it was close enough for him to feel like he was part of his own
care and could make decisions in his own best interest.

I began by telling him how our bodies turn food into energy.

Whatever we eat, we chew up food and swallow it. Once it's in the stomach, our bodies turn that food into sugar. Everything we eat gets turned
into sugar. Then the sugar goes from our stomach into our bloodstream.
Our bloodstream carries the sugar to all the parts of our body—our heart,
our lungs, our brain—until the sugar gets to the cells of our bodies. This is
where the problem comes in. The sugar can't go from the blood into our
cells on its own. It needs help. And the help it needs is insulin. Everybody's
body makes insulin. I think the fact that our own bodies make insulin is
news to most people.

Insulin floats around in the blood, and when it comes upon sugar, it
grabs hold of it and pushes it into the cells. Once the sugar is in the cells,
they are able to turn the sugar into energy, and we live off this energy. But
this is where the problem is. Diabetes is a disease in which something is
wrong with the body's insulin.

After explaining all this, I told Roger, "It just isn't doing the job. And we
know that because when the nurse pricked your finger, she was measuring
how much sugar was in your blood. Normally, that number should be between 70 and 110 early in the morning before you eat."

In Roger's case, it was 323. By any measure, that is way too high.

Roger was following me closely as I explained to him my simplified view
of diabetes. I could tell he really wanted to understand. I continued.

"So," I asked him, "what can we do to fix this problem?"

He was eager to hear my answer.

"Let's say that I am trying to dig a hole out behind our clinic, and I hire
a man to do the job, and I think he will do a good job. Only it turns out he
is lazy. He is just piddling around. How can I get my hole dug?"

Roger was thinking.

"Well," I continued, "one thing I could do is hire several more lazy men.
They might all be lazy, but if I get enough of them working they will eventually dig my hole."

Roger could see how that might work.

"This is what happens when we give you pills. In some ways what we are doing is saying that your own body's insulin is lazy. The pills are telling your body to make more insulin, and even though the insulin is lazy, if we get enough of it into your bloodstream, we can get the job done." (My analogy is not exactly right, but it is close.)

"What, however, are we to do if the men are not just lazy but they quit and lie down on the job? When will I get my hole dug?"

Roger was fully with me. "You'll never get it dug," he declared.

"Exactly. In that case," I said, "the best plan is to go hire a good woman and let her dig the hole."

Roger laughed.

"That is what happens when we have to give people insulin shots. In fact, this is why we started you on insulin, because it was looking like your own body's insulin had quit."

Roger seemed to understand, and it was clear he wanted to know more.

"Roger, diabetes is a complicated disease. The more you know, the better off you will be. You need to make yourself an expert in diabetes. It doesn't do you that much good for me to know all about diabetes. We will teach you if you want to be in control of your own future."

A tear came into the corner of his eye. "Doc, I am so sorry I called you an asshole. I just didn't want to seem so dumb."

I wanted to come closer and hug him, but because of our COVID-19 protocols, I had to just acknowledge that I understood. We were finally heading down a good path. But from this point on, it wasn't going to be me, the doctor, who would help Roger, but our dietician and health coach who would be walking this journey with him.

"Roger, the pills and insulin will help you, but there is so much you can do to help yourself. This all begins with food being turned into sugar, but all food isn't equal. Our dietician will be calling you, and the two of you will work on the best way for you to eat healthy food going forward, and one of our health coaches will be working with you on a plan for exercise, caring for your spirit, and a lot of other ways to get this under control."

In our work at Church Health, we have health coaches embedded into our clinics who work with patients like Roger on behavioral changes that can improve the trajectory of diabetes. We have shown that their work improves outcomes better than all the new drugs to treat diabetes that are advertised on TV.

These days, every other commercial advertises a new diabetic drug that claims to lower hemoglobin A1c. While these drugs do have their place, their benefit comes at quite a price, and that benefit is not nearly as powerful as the happy people in the commercials want you to believe. Most of the new drugs claim to lower hemoglobin A1c by between 0.5 and 1.5.

A few years ago, we began looking closely at what we could do at Church Health to help our patients better manage chronic diseases like diabetes and hypertension, which often occur together and result in people taking multiple prescriptions—or *not* taking them if they can't afford them. We have the resources of a wellness center, health coaches, a teaching kitchen, a behavioral health clinic, an optometry clinic, a dental clinic, and our medical clinics. We value quality improvement.

What could we do better for patients with diabetes?

We bore down on the question and created a system that didn't depend on which provider a patient saw. If a patient had A1c that indicated prediabetes, out-of-control blood sugar with A1c above 7 or 8, or serious numbers above even that—like Roger's were—patients went into an organized system that addressed each level of disease. Now providers had an entire care team to work with. No matter which provider a patient saw or which health coach the patient worked with, standard processes kicked in. This allowed us to document everything that happened, evaluate, and improve.

The result was regular counseling with a health coach led to lowering hemoglobin A1c by 2. That was *without* the addition of the very expensive new medicines that only lowered hemoglobin A1c by 0.5 to 1.5 on their own. The health coaches are also able to give people a sense of agency that pills never will. Many patients can reach their goals and manage their blood sugar levels by understanding their lives as a whole rather than thinking a pill will do all the work. This is a much better way of practicing medicine.

In my years at Church Health, I've seen more patients than I can count with diabetes, hypertension, and heart disease—all chronic conditions that can be prevented in many cases by a better understanding of the difference nutrition and movement can make. As we've demonstrated with our work with diabetes, for many people, better nutrition and movement can make enough difference to avoid years of medications that don't bring as much improvement as healthier living.

I've also reminded a lot of church groups that the least healthy meal people eat all week is often right there at church—favorite potluck dishes or recipes made for a crowd that are full of fat or sugar or sodium. Churches that take on some responsibility for the health of the sheep in their own flocks is a practical way to make a difference. Gathering for shared meals has so many benefits, but we can do this without undercutting people's hard-fought efforts to make better choices or contributing to a culture that suggests they don't have the agency to manage their own health. No one in the congregation with hypertension or diabetes or heart disease is the only one. "I really shouldn't" doesn't seem to stop people from eating church food.

So why not improve church food? It's a challenge worth considering.

Open Arms

Across the country, nurses have found a key role for themselves in promoting prevention and health education through the auspices of the church. Fran Martin became an RN in 1970, was one of the first clinical nurse specialists in Texas, worked in intensive care units, advocated for public health policy, and taught for years at University of Texas with a focus on prevention. She always said that when she retired from University of Texas Arlington College of Nursing, she wanted to work at their free clinic. Instead, through discussions in her church, Fran became convinced she was called to start a clinic that focused primarily on prevention and management of chronic disease. With the commitment of the trustees from her church and a slew of volunteer health professionals and administrative volunteers and interpreters, Open Arms Health Clinic opened in 2011.

At the heart of the practice are ten-week educational classes that patients sign a contract to attend. If for some reason a patient falls off the wagon in attending, they have, in Fran's words, a "come-to-Jesus" meeting to get refocused. It wasn't always this way. Using effective health-promotion strategies based on studies done by Harvard and Stanford has influenced their approach: "This is what you need to be healthy. We'll help you, but you have to take part. If you're not going to do it, move over and make room for someone who wants to." With the contracts for how they expect patients to participate in learning to manage their own chronic diseases, compliance dramatically improved, jumping from 40 percent to 80 percent in the first cycle of the new method.

Fran does this with open arms as part of a church ministry because she is committed to caring for the whole person. Health is part of what the church should be about.

When the COVID-19 pandemic first started, one of Fran's patients contracted the virus, and he was afraid he would get in trouble for not showing up for class. He made sure to call and explain. This is a reflection of how meaningful the wellness classes have become.

Open Arms receives ongoing support from the church as part of their outreach to the community. While Fran is a nurse administrator of a medical clinic open for set hours each week and serving a population base, nurses working in churches in congregational settings also focus on prevention through the movement known as faith community or parish nurses. This idea movement began in the 1970s by a Lutheran minister named Granger Westberg. Westberg believed that nurses working in faith communities could both improve health outcomes and also help people of faith be more faithful to the call God sets before us all to care for our bodies as well as our spirits. Through what is now known as the Westberg Institute for Faith Community Nursing, nursing schools and health-care systems around the world have trained over fifteen thousand nurses to do this work of caring for the whole person. In addition to working in churches, synagogues, mosques, and community centers, faith community nurses work in creative settings, such as Stone Mountain Park, Dollywood, and for the Harlem Globetrotters. It is clear that the practice of prevention in conjunction with faith communities and community resources has a wide array of applications that are not well-known but have the potential to lead people to healthy change.

Heal the City

Heal the City Free Clinic, founded in 2014, is a growing ministry serving the San Jacinto neighborhood of greater Amarillo, Texas. The idea of Heal the City came to Dr. Alan Keister after he traveled on medical missions and began to see his own city as a mission field. Dr. Keister and a group of volunteers started hosting health screenings to provide much-needed medical services and gauge community support for a clinic.

After the idea of Heal the City formed, it was only natural that a congregation step in to provide a critical partnership and get the free clinic on its feet. Just when leadership started to wonder about expansion, a friend of Heal the City mentioned that the neighborhood YMCA was being sold and a building was still available. This building, 22,000 square feet in total, provided essential space for the fast-growing clinic.

In the beginning, Heal the City focused on acute care. But the comprehensive and continuity-of-care piece was missing, and they wanted to do more for patients with chronic diseases. Heal the City started putting together a chronic-care program called Shalom. They chose this term because they wanted the program to encompass complete wellness and flourishing, just as the word indicates. Shalom started by focusing on patients suffering from a chronic disease—such as diabetes—who would benefit from education, continuity of care, and expanded services.

The emphasis on chronic diseases paid off. In the first cohort of Shalom patients with complete data, participants lost an average of 1.7 pounds per month. Of those with diabetes, 16 percent achieved control of their diabetes, and of those with high blood pressure, 43 percent lowered their blood pressure to normal levels. By sitting around a table asking how they could move deeper into whole-person health, Heal the City created a program affecting not only the health of their patients, but also of the greater Amarillo community.

The Heal the City Shalom Chronic Care Program continues to grow due to the number of patients seen through the acute care clinic. As of October 2021, there were 511 individual chronically ill patients enrolled. Shalom patients receive primary care services from one of four nurse practitioners, prescription medications from an on-site class A pharmacy, and routine diagnostic labs. Additional services include vision, dental, mental health, case management, spiritual care, nutrition education, and outside specialty referrals as necessary. As a part of Shalom compliance, patients attend fitness and education classes. In November 2021, Heal the City celebrated the grand opening of the Faith In Transformation (FIT) Center. FIT Center wellness coaches and community volunteers provide class instruction. The goal of the dedicated space is to educate, empower, and encourage patients in their health journeys. Coupling the wellness component with the medical services is proving to be transformational for Shalom patients.

Efforts like Heal the City exist all over, so how can a congregation rally around ministries that are fighting for better holistic health? Besides wrapping your arms around local ministries financially, here are some practical ideas.

- **Offer space.** Many congregations have great space. Can you partner with a ministry that needs extra square footage to carry out its mission?
- **Offer volunteer hours.** Write birthday cards for people who receive services from the ministry, be available to pray during open hours, send encouragement cards to follow up on people you meet, or help organize supplies. You don't need clinical experience to have something to offer a health ministry.
- **Offer meals.** A meal that serves all volunteers during designated open hours of a health ministry will go a long way to sustaining a busy clinical team and those who support them.
- **Offer translation.** If you speak a language other than English used by patients the health ministry serves, write cards for patients, help with paperwork, or find out what it would take to be able to offer translation during clinical services.

The Story in Numbers

Chronic diseases should be front and center in our health-care efforts. Six in ten Americans live with at least one chronic disease—such as heart disease, hypertension, obesity, or diabetes. A quarter of us have two or more, and chronic disease leads to seven in ten deaths.[1] Seventy-five percent of our health-care spending goes toward chronic diseases—and that number rises to 83 percent when we look at the underserved population insured by Medicaid who tend to have multiple risks because of the socioeconomic factors that swirl in their lives and may delay regular care or make it spotty.[2]

Yet our health-care dollars focused on treating chronic disease make a difference. Among the uninsured, 38.4 percent have not seen a physician

even once in the previous twelve months, and 19.6 percent have not received any treatment for a chronic disease in the last year. Among those
insured by Medicaid, these numbers drop to 8.2 percent and 4.5 percent.
People with Medicaid have 8.4 times greater odds of making one or more
visits for chronic disease than the uninsured. Breaking it down even further, people with hypertension who are insured by Medicaid have only a
17 percent chance of making one or fewer visits to a provider, compared to
60 percent for those who are uninsured.[3] The uninsured have a 50 percent
chance of having no source of regular health care, versus 12 percent for
those with insurance.[4] At least one study of sudden death among working-
age adults leads to the conclusion that undiagnosed chronic diseases in
people without insurance contributes to these deaths.[5] For most people,
chronic diseases can be treated and managed long before reaching this
serious stage. Access to regular care is key.

Appreciating God's Gifts

Understanding what it means to be well in body and spirit and developing a
lifestyle that focuses on what works, not on what is broken—that's the heart
of prevention and managing chronic diseases that have become rampant
in an increasingly sedentary culture.

Technology absorbs the time, talent, and resources we need for keeping
us healthy. We too often wait until we break, rather than looking ahead to
prevent the breaks. Take childhood obesity as an example. It's frequently
in the news, and it should be. We are raising a generation of kids who go
home from school, sit on the couch, play on the Xbox, and snack on food
that offers no nutrition. These obese children *will* be adults who have hypertension, diabetes, heart attacks, and trouble finding employment. But
we must do more than talk about it and look at pictures of sedentary children eating processed food. If we dedicate resources to fighting obesity
through preventing it in the first place, we can make a far greater difference
in the health of a generation than will ever come from developing a next
generation MRI or new drugs for erectile dysfunction. Because of our love
affair with technology, we are failing to give children hope for their own
futures. While we debate how to give them access to technology in the
event that their bodies break down—and they will—we overlook giving

them the love and joy and self-understanding essential to real health for the whole person.

While we're at the top of the chart when it comes to technology, we're at the bottom of the chart when it comes to prevention. What might happen to our health if we shifted at least some portion of our reliance from fixing what breaks to being connected in faith to the way God created us?

A woman who suffered for twelve years with a continuous illness followed Jesus. She went to lots of doctors. The Talmud, an ancient Jewish teaching text, contains medicines and treatments prescribed for the kind of illness the woman had, and no doubt she tried them all in twelve years. But she got worse, not better. Now she was ready to bring faith into the story. This woman heard about Jesus, but she didn't want to be too much trouble. She thought, "If I but touch his clothes, I will be made well" (Mark 5:28). Her faith gave her hope when nothing else did. When she managed to graze Jesus's clothing as he walked by, she "felt in her body that she was healed of her disease."

Despite the woman's subtle action of touching the cloak of a man in motion, Jesus knew something happened, and he was determined to find out who touched him. The woman was petrified, but she told the truth. Jesus said, "Daughter, your faith has made you well; go in peace, and be healed of your disease" (Mark 5:34).

Faith, healing, peace, freedom from suffering—all in one brief encounter. Jesus did not separate faith from health. Jesus interacted with the whole person. If we begin to interact with ourselves as whole people, perhaps we will also begin to interact with others as whole people.

And then our perspectives on tackling chronic diseases might really change.

For Reflection

1. Have you ever had an encounter with a physician that was as direct in tone as Roger's getting a reality check about his diabetes? If so, how did that make you feel? If not, how do you think you would respond?

2. Do you have any chronic health conditions or family history that means you should be mindful of risks? How are you responding to these condi-

tions in your life? Do you feel that you're managing well, or do you wish you had better support?

3. How do you feel about shared meals and your own goals and eating habits? Do you make exceptions to your goals for shared meals, such as church potlucks or going out to lunch with friends, or do you try to make choices that keep you on track?

EIGHT

WHAT'S ON YOUR MIND IS IN YOUR BODY

Zyanya has long black hair with dark brown eyes set in her deep-hued, round face, the features of someone indigenous to Central America. Over time I have come to recognize physical features of people from different parts of Latin America, and I suspected Zyanya had Mayan heritage. When I suspect someone is from an indigenous people, I know there is a good chance Spanish is not the person's first language. Often our Spanish interpreters have trouble fully understanding someone whose native language is a derivative of Mayan. Thankfully, Zyanya seemed to also speak Spanish well.

When I see a woman from a rural part of Central America, I worry almost immediately that she left her home because of a violent past. Many women like Zyanya left because of fear of gangs or sexual violence. I have gotten to where I assume something like that is in their past and usually don't explore very deeply why they left. My assumption is the answer would be a very painful memory.

In talking to Zyanya through an interpreter, I learned I was right that she was from Honduras. Like most Latina women from Central America who are our patients, Zyanya was working as a housekeeper.

These days, in Memphis, we have become a trusted place for immigrants to receive health care. It took years for this to become true, however. When Church Health began in 1987, our patient population was roughly 50 percent Black and 50 percent White. There was a fairly small immigrant population in a city divided along racial lines for its entire existence. During the 1990s, however, the Mexican population began to slowly grow. As migrant and construction workers appeared, the women who came with them began cleaning houses. We would occasionally see someone in our clinic who spoke Spanish, and, thankfully, two of our providers were fluent. But we had no one on the telephones or on our nursing staff who was fluent, and I couldn't get past "buenos dias."

I could sense, though, that we needed to reach out to the Latinx community to tell them we were here for them. Mary Braza, a family doctor on our staff who spoke Spanish, agreed to regularly appear on the Spanish-speaking radio station to talk about health-care issues. Then Claudia, a native of Colombia whose daughter was a patient at St. Jude's Children's Research Hospital, wanted to volunteer as a translator for patients who spoke Spanish. It made sense to see how she did.

Still, the number of Spanish-speaking patients we saw only trickled in. I couldn't at first understand why. We provided quality care at a very affordable price, and we were sympathetic to their cause. What more was there for us to do?

It took time and much frustration on my part, but slowly the numbers began to grow. Claudia became an employee. We started hiring other Spanish speakers from Mexico and Central America. At some point we seemed to cross the Rubicon. We became a trusted place. It wasn't just that we would not turn undocumented immigrants into the authorities but that we would take the time to understand their concerns and the challenges they faced. Mary Nell Ford, a Johns Hopkins-trained internist, took it on herself to learn Spanish. And she told me one day, "People ask, 'Whatever happened to the American family, where the father works two jobs, the mom stays home to take care of the children, and they go to church every Sunday?'" She continued, "That family still exists. It just so happens that they speak Spanish."

I knew she was right.

Our challenge began to be not how to get people to come to the doctor when they were sick but to help them understand what it meant to have a family doctor. We could help them focus on living a healthy life, not just wait until something was broken. Few of those we saw from Mexico and Central America had ever had a regular doctor. And they were averse to anything other than paying their own way as they went, so the huge cost of most medical procedures meant they wouldn't even start the process of seeing a doctor unless the reason for care was urgent and unavoidable. We continue to struggle to get many of our Latinx patients to understand that we will care for them without that care costing all the money they have saved this month to send back home to their families.

When I first walked into the room, I could feel a sense of sadness in Zyanya. There was no smile as she sat in the exam room chair. By any measure a pretty woman in her early forties, she somehow seemed older. As I introduced myself to her and began asking questions, she looked at the floor and gave cryptic answers. I tried to find out a little about her, but she was not forthcoming.

"How long have you been in Memphis?" It was a simple question.

Her answer was confusing. "I have been here with my family."

I tried again to make contact. "What kind of work do you do?"

"I clean houses."

My other attempts to connect did not make much headway. Finally I asked, "What can I do to help you today?"

There was a pause, then she began quietly to tell Teresita, the interpreter, why she had come. Zyanya and Teresita had a long conversation back and forth. I knew Teresita was having trouble getting her to be clear.

Finally, Teresita said to me, "She says there is a problem 'down there.'"

That meant this was a gynecological issue.

After more unhelpful conversation, I surmised that Zyanya was having pelvic pain and I needed to do a pelvic exam. Zyanya would need to get undressed, and I would need to look and examine her with my hands. I intended for the words I used and the way I spoke to be as gentle as possible. Still Zyanya paused.

"I can only help you if I can examine you," I said.

She nodded, and I gave her a gown to put on and stepped outside.

While we were waiting for her to get undressed, I asked Teresita if she sensed something not right with Zyanya. She replied, "I know she is scared, but I'm not sure why."

In doing her exam, I did not find anything abnormal. When I asked her to point to the pain, she could only tell me that the pain was all over. When I finished, I told her she could get dressed. Back in the room again, I worked to get a better feel for when the pain began and to better understand its nature. The story slowly unraveled.

"When did you start having this pain?"

"Six weeks ago."

I asked about her periods and everything else I could think of. Nothing made sense.

"Did something happen to you?" I had begun to have my worries. I kept pulling in a way I felt was slowly, in a small way, trying to win her trust.

Again, she and Teresita had a long back and forth discussion. I could only make out an occasional word. And then Zyanya began to cry unstoppably.

Teresita tried to translate to me through the tears as I moved closer to offer some form of comfort even though I didn't know what I was comforting her about.

Teresita began. "She was working at a house she has worked at for several years in Collierville." (This is an affluent suburb of Memphis.) "The owners of the house are having extensive renovations done, which made it hard for Zyanya to get her work done. Normally the woman owner of the house is there when Zyanya is working, but she had stepped out to do some errands. There was a crew of men left in the house alone with Zyanya. For several weeks they had been making remarks to Zyanya. Since she does not speak English, she did not know what they were saying. She knew they were coming on to her, so she just tried to ignore it. This day, they became more aggressive. She tried to just go on about her work, but two of the men came up to her and cornered her. She turned away, but one grabbed her arm. Zyanya tried to pull away but to no avail. The second one began kissing her."

From there it turned into a horrible nightmare. It took thirty minutes for both of them to rape her. Her clothes were torn, and she was humiliated. She couldn't believe that God would let this happen to her.

She grabbed what she could of her things and fled from the house. Lost and broken, she didn't know what to do or who to turn to. She couldn't call the police. I suspect she thought they would have asked to see her papers before listening to her story about the rape. At least I want to believe that, but I can't be certain. I can imagine her fear of being deported and how it would impact her children overrode all reasonable thought to call the police and ask for their help. She would rather suffer the trauma at hand than the trauma to come.

After the attack, Zyanya couldn't stop crying. She went home and decided not to tell anyone. Unmarried and with grown children who didn't live with her, she lived with her brother and his family. Her tears kept flowing. Despite the challenges she faced back in Honduras and in coming to the United States, she has always been very religious, always believed that "God will watch over me." Only now her deep faith was shaken.

Since coming to Memphis, almost all her social connections had come from her church. She went every Sunday. In church she felt God's love at every turn. The rape, though, made her unsure of God's love.

Feeling desperate, she turned to the pastor of the church for help. She reluctantly went to tell him what had happened. What Zyanya told Teresita he said was, "You must keep working at that house because you must confront your demons."

And so, that is what she had been doing. She kept returning to the house as though nothing had happened. Thankfully the men who raped her had not been around, but every time she stepped into the house she could feel their presence. Her pulse would quicken and her mind returned to the unthinkable.

It had been six weeks since the rape when she came to our walk-in clinic. She had friends who are our patients, so she decided to see if we could help her with the pain she was continuing to have in her pelvis.

After hearing the gist of what had happened, I was fairly clear about the cause of her pain. I made sure I tested her for sexually transmitted infections, but the source of her pelvic pain was not physical. It was because the men had crushed her heart. No technology is available to detect the source of her distress, and no pills would heal the wound.

I also knew that my giving her an extra fifteen minutes of my great wisdom would not be of much help. I suspected I reminded her more of the men who raped her or of the pastor who gave her horrendous advice than I did of someone who could lead her out of the valley of the shadow of death.

What I did next, I believe, helped ease her pain. I called for one of our Spanish-speaking counselors to come see her.

Half of the people who come to primary care doctors like me have no physical medical problem. They are there because of their mental and emotional health needs. These days, people come to the doctor for reasons they used to visit the priest or pastor. Why is that? It is partly because people have decreased trust in the clergy and partly because clergy are less well trained or available to deal with matters of the heart. Unfortunately, physicians are equally ill-equipped to care for matters of the spirit. We are so focused on physical ailments that we can't see the spiritual dis-ease people have. We are so dependent on technology that we assume our diagnostic testing will reveal the cause of all human suffering. But I could have MRIed Zyanya's heart all day long and I never would have uncovered the slow bleeding of her damaged soul.

On that first day of meeting her, Stephanie, the counselor who began seeing her, was able to make a connection and help Zyanya start down a healing path. Six weeks later Zyanya came back for a follow-up with me on her pelvic pain. When I walked in the door, the heaviness in the room was much lighter.

Teresita was again my interpreter. "It is good to see you. How are you doing?"

For the first time, Zyanya looked at me and smiled. She is a beautiful woman who has endured much. "I am better."

"How is your pain?" There were two sources of pain: her pelvis and her heart.

She assumed I was only asking about her pelvic pain. "It is gone," she seemed happy to tell me.

"I am so glad." I then turned to the most important issue. "How is it going with Stephanie?"

Zyanya paused. "Good." But her smile was gone.

I had been able to read the notes Stephanie had written in her chart after their counseling sessions. I could tell there was much for them to discuss beyond the rape. What had happened to Zyanya back in Honduras was almost as traumatic. In addition, the ordeal of coming to and living in the United States was immense. Still, Zyanya was pushing on.

"I hope you will keep seeing Stephanie," I said with a smile and as much encouragement as I could. I also had to say, "If other things come up you can always come talk to us about how you should handle them. I am not sure your pastor gave you the best advice, but I am sure he wanted you to continue to feel God's love."

I felt what he had said was about the worst advice he could have given her, but I also knew that the church was one of the few sources of comfort she had. It is just not a perfect world or church.

Since then, Zyanya has continued to see Stephanie. She found a new cleaning job. I have seen her a couple of times for small medical problems. I know we have not solved her problem. Such immense mental health wounds do not heal easily, but for now, her life is better.

Mental Health in the Church

People facing mental health issues are in the church, as we see from Zyanya's story. We also see from Zyanya's story that the church is not always well prepared to care for mental illness or emotional distress. Often we don't realize the prevalence of mental health concerns in the church—the same as in the general population—or the urgency to minister to them.

"She came looking for help on a Sunday morning." Bishop William Young, twenty years after the fact, still feels the remorse of wishing he and others in the church had better understood the crisis level of the woman's grief. Instead, he told her to come back the next morning and he would try and help. Many pastors just want to get through Sunday.

She did return the next morning—at 6:30.

"She went and stood under the cross at the altar and pulled out a pistol and shot herself," Bishop Young said. It was devastating for him and the congregation.

The experience led to a twenty-year mission to address suicide in the Black church. Bishop William Young has been a chaplain at Western State Mental Health Center in Bolivar, Tennessee, and a chaplain at Methodist Health Systems in Memphis. He was well qualified to lead such a charge. Together with his wife, Rev. Dianne P. Young, he hosted the first National Suicide and the Black Church Conference in Memphis in 2003 and continues to speak around the country. Tragedy can be galvanizing, and ultimately it may open awareness and opportunity for the church to take a leading role.

Matt Russell's personal experience was galvanizing. Matt grew up in an evangelical Christian family in Dallas, Texas. When he was twelve, his mother became sick. In the church, people accused her of unconfessed sin and being an unsubmissive wife. It turned out she had a brain tumor.

Matt felt that he was part of the problem. He thought, There's something wrong and I need to do something. The church didn't seem the place to help him cope. He managed by reaching out for "substances and processes." He created his own anxiety-management system for which he had a "high bottom," meaning he hid his substance abuse well. He used anything that would numb him physically and allow him to cope with his overwhelming experiences, first with his mother's death and then the challenges of life. He developed a process that would never leave a trail. No one knew, and as a result he felt constant shame. In other words, he became a high-functioning addict.

Despite all his struggles, Matt sought to become a pastor and went to seminary. He was in endless conflict over the God he had been taught growing up—judgmental, harsh, demanding—and the God he had come to know—loving, kind, accepting. The disconnect led to a crisis of faith.

At twenty-seven, in his first appointment as a United Methodist minister, Matt met an Alcoholics Anonymous "old timer." It was a burning bush experience where he felt God was truly present. This led him to go to treatment, where he experienced confession not as shame but as joy. It was liberating. He saw God—YHWH—as one where "something is happening here."

When Matt returned to the church, he asked the senior pastor, Jim Jackson, to let him interview people who had left the church and ask them why. His goal was to start a congregation for people who hate church. What he found was a recurring theme of people who had found their spirits touched through AA and the recovery community, just as he had. Through recovery, people had experienced a vital spirituality.

Why should a mental and behavioral health issue be causing people to leave the church and find renewal elsewhere? But it was.

The church for people who hate church took on the name Mercy Street. It began with about sixty people the first time they met, most of them in recovery. And then it grew. And it grew.

No matter how people had been harmed, they found a source of solace in Mercy Street.

Joe had recently been released from prison. He had every intention of stealing a car when he was invited to Mercy Street. As he entered the building, a woman asked, "Is this your first time here?"

He told her, "Yes."

She then said, "Come sit with me."

He did. He got up to go to the bathroom with the intent to sneak out. She got up and went with him. And she waited. He would later say, "She was like a booger I couldn't get off of my finger." By the third week of going, he joined the church.

While Matt was the pastor, the regular attendance grew to around a thousand people. Matt sees what happened in the same light as the prophet Isaiah: "A new thing is happening here." Matt believes that "the spirit of God wants to do things like this all the time." Matt saw Mercy Street as "building what I needed when my mom got sick." It isn't built on a set of beliefs you are expected to follow; it is built on what God is doing in the world now, and God invites Christians to it. Almost one-third of those who attend Mercy Street are "normies"—people not in recovery in any formal sense but who are drawn to the ministry because of what it says to them about the goodness of God.

Matt left Mercy Street in 2008 for other activist ministries in Houston, and the church continues to thrive as a place that leads people to be strong in the broken places.

We can face galvanizing events and hear God's call for not only our own mental health but the health of others, or we can pretend those things don't happen among God's people.

But they do happen, and they happen among God's people. The call to heal includes mental and behavioral health.

The Story in Numbers

Access to mental health services is a significant problem across the United States. This problem is worse if you belong to one of any number of vulnerable populations affected by poverty. For instance, one-fifth of children have mental health issues, but only 20 percent of those children receive care from a mental health specialist.[1] However, less than 15 percent of children who live in poverty and need mental health services receive them, and an even lower number complete treatment plans. Children don't receive care for a variety of reasons. The wait time for an appointment at a mental health clinic can be quite long, and they don't always have flexible hours to accommodate variable shifts of parents who have little control of assigned work hours. Some mothers fear anyone in the household being labeled "crazy" and having children removed from their care.[2]

Like any health care, a lack of insurance increases the vulnerability of not being treated for mental health needs. Forty-two percent of people who live at lower incomes see cost and poor insurance as a top barrier to accessing mental health services, and 25 percent report choosing between getting mental health treatment and paying for daily necessities. In rural areas, the round-trip drive to receive treatment is more than an hour for 46 percent of residents. While mental health issues affect all socioeconomic, racial, and ethnic groups, someone in a household earning less than $35,000 a year is four times more likely to report being "nervous" and five times as likely to report being "sad" all or most of the time compared to households with incomes above $100,000.[3] Millions of Americans have a mental illness and are uninsured. Over 57 percent of people in the United States with a mental illness have gone without treatment. Twenty-six million people report going untreated because of lack of insurance, shortage of psychiatrists willing to treat someone without insurance or to take insurance, shortage of outpatient or inpatient care appropriate to the need, and disconnect between primary care clinics and behavioral-care services.[4]

Perhaps one of the most unmentionable realities of mental health care is how it negatively impacts other health care. People with severe mental illness die fifteen to thirty years younger than those who do not have these illnesses. People with mental health illness are less likely to get cardiac catheterization when they have chest pain, less likely to get appropriate care to manage diabetes, less likely to get screening and treatment for cancer—the health care most of us expect that could help prevent or manage chronic disease for longer life.[5]

The undocumented immigrants among us find themselves vulnerable in their mental health as well as their physical health. Nearly a quarter of them have experienced some mental health disorder; 14 percent have major depressive disorder; 8 percent have a panic disorder; 7 percent have an anxiety disorder; over 80 percent report a history of trauma; 47 percent report significant psychological distress; 59 percent experience domestic violence; 56 percent have witnessed violence; and the experience of post-traumatic stress disorder among undocumented women is four times higher than for other women in the United States—34 percent versus 9.7 percent. The experience does not wane over time.[6]

Children, people with low incomes who know they are struggling, people with severe mental illness, immigrants—these are only a few vulnerable populations. I have no doubt we could isolate more and demonstrate other risks. We have to work harder at removing stigmas, removing obstacles, and believing in the health of the whole person because that is who God created us to be.

Healing Partnerships

In Luke 10, we read the story of Jesus sending seventy of his followers out in pairs. Jesus sent them out to announce that the kingdom of God—God's sovereign rule—is here and now. Jesus gave specific instructions on how his followers should respond if people received them in peace and what to do if they met hostility. At the heart of those specific, explicit instructions, Jesus said, "Cure the sick who are there, and tell them, 'The kingdom of God has come near to you'" (Luke 10:9).

Though we think of ourselves as Jesus's followers—and thus he is the leader—in this instance, he sent the seventy on "ahead of him in pairs to every town and place where he himself intended to go" (Luke 10:1). But Jesus did not go at that time. He commissioned those who had been learning from him to do the same work he had been doing of preaching and demonstrating the kingdom and gave specific instructions to heal as part of their announcement of the kingdom. Clearly he expected them to heal. He expected them to do as they saw him do over and over. They should have expected to see God's kingdom's power working through their actions. And when the seventy followers returned, they said, "Lord, in your name even the demons submit to us!" (Luke 10:17). They were perhaps astonished at their own message of the kingdom.

In the realm of healing mental and behavioral wounds and diseases, taking on the healing ministry of Jesus matters for caring for whole persons. We all have our "demons," emotional wounds, traumas, seasons of better or worse mental health. Some among us fight harder against the substances and processes that keep them from true wholeness, and they need the rest of us beside them with assurances that the gospel is for the whole person, body and spirit—even crushed spirits. Just as Jesus's disciples went out in partnership and were astonished at what became of their ministry, perhaps we too would be astonished at the healing that would come from kingdom partnerships between the mental health community and the faith community if we faced our galvanizing events as opportunities to learn and engage.

For Reflection

1. Zyanya's story is one that is difficult to turn our hearts away from. At the same time, it's often difficult to know how to help someone experiencing circumstances that threaten their mental health. What makes you feel most uncomfortable in situations involving mental illness? What helps you find ways to respond positively?

2. Think about your own experience of mental and emotional health and the church. Has the church been a place you could count on for support and understanding, or has it been a place where you felt you had to hide your "weaknesses"? What lasting impact has this experience left on you?

3. Can you think of a person in your own life who models for you compassionate and practical ways to respond to someone who is experiencing mental or behavioral illness? What have you learned from this person?

NINE

ECHOES OF GOD'S LOVE

In the summer of 1989, about two years after Church Health opened, I met Mary Leslie Simpson when I was speaking at a conference in Nashville. Although in the same state, the distance from Memphis to Knoxville, where Mary Leslie lived, is almost the same as Knoxville to Washington, DC, and culturally the two cities are a world apart.

Mary Leslie was a committed Catholic and enamored with the idea of faith-based health care. I was at the time only thirty-five years old and she wasn't much older. She had no health-care background, but I could feel her passion. She came to Memphis to see our work when Church Health was in just one small building with three exam rooms. Immediately she itched to do something similar in Knoxville and returned to connect to Catholic Charities there. After talking to the broader faith community in Knoxville, she asked me to come speak to those she had interested. She was hard to resist.

By the fall, Mary Leslie was on her way. She was a master at approaching people in such a way that they couldn't turn away from helping her cause. On March 6, 1991, Interfaith Health Clinic opened its doors. When I read their mission statement and understood their vision, it was almost identical to Church Health. Now for thirty years, Interfaith has done this work with over four hundred thousand clinical visits.

I didn't realize it at the time, but Mary Leslie's request to learn about what Church Health was doing would only be the first of many.

From Insurance to Safety Nets

Why was there such a need, even thirty or forty years ago, for clinics like Church Health and Interfaith?

It hasn't always been this way. In the early twentieth century, the Social Gospel movement argued that the new science and new medical techniques that emerged during the late nineteenth century should be made available for all Americans. The power of this idea led to the building of church-owned hospitals across the United States. Hospitals with the names Baptist, Methodist, St. Francis, and many more sprouted up with the desire for faith communities to live the biblical mandate to care for the body but also to assure that the new medicine would be made available to all, including the poor who were sick.

The practice of medicine was seen as a helping profession far more than a business. Doctors might be paid in chickens, and care was often bartered for what people could offer in exchange. Doctors expected a third of their practice would be charity care. It was the nature of the profession.

In 1929 Blue Cross began in Texas to help people afford the services of a group of hospitals if the time came that they needed them. A decade later, Blue Shield formed in California as a way to prepay the services of physicians. As the plans spread across states, people would often buy both. (The two did not merge until 1982.) Generally, there wasn't that much health care to insure because there wasn't that much health care to buy in the first place, so costs were not outrageous when the plans began.

World War II changed US health care. During the war, with so many citizens in the armed forces, the nation faced a labor shortage. However, the federal government was concerned that businesses competing for workers by increasing wages would cause inflation to get out of hand, and President Roosevelt signed an executive order freezing wages. To compete for quality employees, new business strategies emerged. One of these was providing benefits to workers. Health care was a private matter until businesses realized guaranteeing employees their health-care costs would be covered was a way around the wage freezes. After the war, in many European countries, the government was the only possible way to provide health care on the devastated continent. In the United States, though, business had already taken on the role of providing health care as a benefit. In the decade from

1940 to 1950, the number of Americans with some kind of insurance went from 9 percent to 50 percent and continued to climb.

Who was left out? The elderly and children of the very poor, two groups not expected to be in the workforce. Then in 1965, President Lyndon Johnson's "war on poverty" led to the creation of Medicare and Medicaid—Medicare for those over 65 and those with disabilities, and Medicaid for poor children and pregnant women.

While there has been much talk in the last thirty years about "health care for all" in the United States, in the late 1960s, the country came close to universal care. Between business coverage, Medicare, and Medicaid, there were few gaps in the system. As a result, all over the country, signs went up in doctors' offices that said, "Payment is expected at the time of service." This was because of the common assumption that every person had some form of health-care coverage. Doctors pulled back on the amount of charity care they offered because it was not needed anymore. Unfortunately, this didn't last very long.

When the tradition of physicians seeing the poor for free began to wane, it fell to the emergency rooms of hospitals to care for the uninsured. For many years the church-owned hospitals readily accepted this challenge, but in the 1970s and 1980s churches began to question the reasoning for their owning hospital systems. This increased as the concept of for-profit hospitals emerged. The Hospital Corporation of America and Tenet Health Care began buying hospitals that were started in the early twentieth century by denominations. Quickly, the not-for-profit community-based and church-owned hospitals were struggling to compete with the for-profit health-care systems who could also care for many low-income people because now Medicare or Medicaid would reimburse them. Margins began to matter in a way they never had before. Caring for the poor became a burden. The message of the gospel Jesus taught was foolhardy by Wall Street standards. Quality health care for the uninsured was becoming a distant memory.

Fairly soon, gaps in coverage appeared even among those who worked, mostly among people working low-wage jobs. The cost of providing health coverage through insurance was a luxury many small employers couldn't—or wouldn't—cover. Mom-and-pop businesses, barely making it financially, remained uninsured. Most service industry jobs were left out. Housekeepers, dishwashers, janitors, lawn-care workers, day care workers, gravedig-gers, and on and on increased the ranks of the uninsured. From 1965 until 1987, when I came to Memphis to start Church Health, the number grew to twenty-seven million uninsured Americans. The number has continued to rise ever since.

ECHO: The Church Health Model

The Church Health model begins with engaging the faith community to do what God calls us to do—care for our bodies as well as our spirits, and to also care for the poor when they are sick. If healing ministry is what God expects of Jesus's followers, then it will always be upon the church both to do the work and find the resources to sustain the ministry. The focus of such church-based ministries should be on where the need is greatest. At Church Health, as at many other clinics following our model, we focus on providing a primary care home for people who are working but neverthe-less remain uninsured.

After Mary Leslie's request to hear about our work when we were barely two years old, inquiries to visit our clinic began to grow. At first it was flattering, but it soon became extremely time-consuming to interrupt our schedule of caring for patients to show individuals around and answer questions and give lengthy explanations. The questions and answers fell into a pattern, and we began holding "replication seminars" for groups representing several potential new or fledgling clinics at a time. In a two-day experience we tried, in an organized way, to answer the questions I wished people would have answered for me when I first started, even the small things. For example, if you are ordering a blood pressure cuff out of a catalogue, do you know what you get? You get a blood pressure cuff. You don't get the bladder you need to inflate it in order to take a patient's blood pressure. That has to be ordered separately. So many pitfalls could be avoided if we just laid out the plan for what it takes to start such an endeavor, from the details of setting up exam rooms to engaging the faith community and finding funding apart from relying on the government.

Quickly, people from all over the country began to come. We standard-ized our presentations, and they kept coming. It was clear there was a hun-ger for doing this type of work. They still come. I am not alone in reading the New Testament and seeing that following Jesus requires a commitment to a healing ministry. The question remains, What does this look like in today's world? Faith-based health clinics modeled after Church Health is one answer to that question.

Interfaith in Knoxville was the first replication clinic to open and be successful. Soon after, both Interfaith Dental and Faith Family Medical Center in Nashville followed. Dr. Tom Underwood had traveled the world doing volunteer dental clinics when he realized that low-income people in his own community of Nashville had dental problems as bad as anything he encountered in the developing world. In 1994, with the help of the Nashville Dental Association and the West End United Methodist Church, Dr. Underwood started a dental clinic with two chairs for the working uninsured. Soon, with the help of Dr. Rhonda Switzer-Nadasdi, the clinic grew dramatically. It built a new building, opened a second location, and now has twenty-six dental operatories to treat thousands of patients every year. Physicians David Gaw and John Lamb were the visionaries behind Faith Family Medical Clinic. Since 2001, Faith Family has been caring for the working uninsured and other underserved Middle Tennesseans.

The challenges in every community to start a faith-based clinic followed the same pattern: developing a broad base of support, designing the scope of service, fundraising, engaging the local health-care and faith communities, and finding those people willing to dedicate their careers to the ministry. To further these goals, Church Health began to partner with a group based in Fort Worth, Texas, named ECHO (Empowering Church Health Outreach), working on similar goals to develop charitable clinics and inspiring faith communities across the United States to develop whole-person health-care ministries for the underserved. ECHO brought a team with decades of experience coaching church-based groups to success in opening charitable clinics. With the support of a Fort Worth philanthropist, John Snyder, ECHO and Church Health set out to grow clinics based on the Church Health model in communities that had the leadership to follow the direction that staff from ECHO set forward.

Now Church Health replication seminars are an opportunity for church and community leaders to not only pick the brains of staff at Church Health but also to encounter the expertise of ECHO to start, grow, and sustain their clinics. For many, the next phase after visiting Church Health is to work with ECHO consultants to identify their own next steps. ECHO provides complimentary assistance for every step, from inspiration to opening a clinic with a solid business plan.

These clinics all emerge once committed leadership catches the spirit of the vision. Since 2015, it has been remarkable to see how deep the desire across the United States is to move from clinics that might have had a vision in the past for a few hours a week in a church basement to establishing well-run, full-time, faith-based clinics. Places like The Well in Cactus, Texas, or Open Arms in Arlington, Texas, or Heal the City in Amarillo, Texas, or Healing Grove in San Jose, California, are part of a larger movement of faith-based clinics that care for both body and spirit without building budget around government funds.

The Story in Numbers

The concept of safety net providers took shape in the 1970s in response to the need to care for the uninsured. Community-based hospitals in large cities, usually affiliated with a medical school, became the provider of care for anyone who was poor. The "doctor's office" became a clinic staffed by young physicians in training or even by medical students. Caring for people with little to no financial resources became a way to learn your trade. Health care in the emergency room was the norm even though no one believed it was a good way to provide health care. It was the last resort.

The federal government also began funding primary care clinics across the country through the Health Resources and Services Administration (HRSA) via the Bureau of Primary Health Care. The law that governs the clinics comes from Section 330 of the Public Health Services Act. Since the 1960s the number of clinics has grown dramatically from only eight clinics to 1,368 Federally Qualified Health Centers (FQHCs) across the country with more than 13,500 service-delivery sites. In the last twenty years, FQHCs have nearly tripled the number of patients they serve to twenty-nine million.[1]

These clinics receive relatively large sums of money from state and federal funds as long as they provide a minimum of care to people who either have Medicaid or Medicare (which not all doctors accept) or are uninsured. Under President Obama, large amounts of money were poured into the Community Health Network through the Affordable Care Act (ACA). New FQHCs emerged designed to care for the expanded number of previously uninsured people newly eligible for Medicaid. A number of these new FQHCs were started and run by people of faith. With new FQHC clinics established, along with the expanded funding for Medicaid in many states, on paper it seemed like the issue of health care for the poor was being solved.

Only, it was not.

Through the Supreme Court's ruling in favor of a case brought by Republicans litigating parts of the Affordable Care Act, a number of states, mostly in the South, never expanded Medicaid rolls the way the ACA intended. Even in states that did expand Medicaid, the scope of the problem of access to quality health care for people living on low incomes continued to grow.

The millions of uninsured, even with Medicaid expansion through the ACA, are only one reason that clinics like Church Health exist. Also, in no federal plan is there willingness to provide access to those who are living and working in the United States but who remain undocumented. Even "Medicare for all" would not make it possible for every poor person in the country to receive care.

In the same decades that FQHCs have grown using taxpayer dollars, free and charitable clinics have sprung up all over the country funded by philanthropy. In the beginning, clinics started by people with good hearts but limited means might offer a clinic in a church basement one night a week staffed with a variety of volunteers. There was never a shortage of patients. Free and charitable clinics have grown with the need, continuing to fill the gap that even well-intended government programs leave and maturing into clinics with more services and more hours.

We mentioned in chapter 2 that these clinics cared for 2.9 million patients in 2019. Even though the COVID-19 pandemic slowed access to care for many of these vulnerable patients, free and charitable clinics added 537,000 new patients in 2020. Of the individuals these clinics care for, 60 percent are employed, but 85 percent are uninsured. While 40 percent of the general US population are racial and ethnic minorities, 64 percent of people who receive care at free and charitable clinics are minorities. We continue to battle health-care disparities.[2]

Throughout this book, you've read stories of people working in free and charitable clinics in communities where access to health care still has many gaps, and I've mentioned ECHO, Empowering Church Health Outreach. These clinics work with free consultants with years of experience to go through a planning process and get them up on their feet and running with the Church Health model of caring for the whole person, addressing the needs of the spirit as well as the body because God created us as whole beings, and operating with a philanthropic model rather than relying on government funding. As of 2021, over ninety clinics are using this model. Together, they care for nearly 270,000 patients through over 830,000 patient visits annually. Eighty percent of ECHO clinics are rooted in faith community initiatives motivated by people of faith caring for the poor who are sick because they believe this is what God calls them to do. They are spread across the United States from Florida to California, from Texas to Wisconsin, from New Jersey to Alabama and Nebraska. These clinics operate with paid physicians, use electronic medical records, and provide comprehensive care. Each year new clinics open by collaborating with the ECHO consulting process. Any community interested in exploring the feasibility of opening a faith-based health-care ministry to care for the whole person can contact ECHO for initial questions and guidance.[3]

From Mississippi to the Bronx to You

Patrick Ball is the son of a family practice physician in rural Mississippi. Tall and lean with graying hair and in his early fifties, his round glasses and gray beard give him a professorial look. He had been practicing medicine in private practice in northern Mississippi for twenty years, but he was ready for a change that would fill something that was missing.

Growing up, Patrick went with his father on rounds where he would hang on every move his father made. His eyes were open and his mind raced with what he saw. "I got to see a lot of suffering that didn't get met." He remembers the challenges he would see among the rural poor of the poorest state in the country.

When he was ten, he was on rounds with his father in a nursing home. He remembers the smell in the halls that day. While his father was writing notes in a patient's chart, he stopped and turned to Patrick and said, "Son, I'm going to tell you the secret to life."

Patrick was all ears. Even at ten he knew that this would be important. His father went on, "You have got to love people."

Patrick was a little disappointed with what his father said. That was it?

After a few minutes his father continued, "Whether you turn out to be a banker, a farmer, or a doctor, loving people is what matters."

For the next forty years, Patrick didn't forget what his father said, but it took that long for him to conclude, "I now get it."

As committed Christians, Patrick and his wife struggled to know how this understanding played out in their lives. Medicine provided a good living financially for their family, but there was more to what they were looking for. He told me, "If you believe there is a God, and God is love, there are things required of you."

Armed with this point of view, Patrick became the first physician for Trinity Health Center in Horn Lake, Mississippi, in a county known to have thirty thousand uninsured residents. His decision was a direct result of having watched his father provide both medical and spiritual care in a small community.

The clinic, nurtured by ECHO's expertise, is a remarkable achievement born out of the desire to work together of two very large churches in the community: Brown Baptist led by Rev. Bartholomew Orr, and Life Fellowship led by Rev. Patrick Conrad. One congregation is historically Black and the other White. Both are committed to taking the gospel seriously on the matter of healing. Together they bought and refurbished a building and committed to working side by side. Dr. Ball is now the physician who will help make their vision come alive to spread Christ's love through quality health care and provide hope and healing to underserved neighbors.

In the Bronx, New York, it is Claudette Phipps and Dr. Deborah Hunter-Brown who have heard the call to start an ECHO clinic. Both grew up in Jamaica but came to the United States in young adulthood. Claudette, a home economics teacher in Jamaica, became a dietician in the United States and moved through a management career in community health centers, including serving as chief development officer for an FQHC. In the last few years, she began wanting more from her work and sought a way to connect her faith to her desire for better health care for those in the Bronx community she had been serving for thirty years. She knew people were still falling through the cracks of the system. By the time Claudette heard about Church Health and came to Memphis for an ECHO replication seminar, she was already looking toward opening a faith-based clinic in the Bronx. Her entire career had prepared her for the moment she now faced. Within three months of the seminar, she had filled out the paperwork to become a 501(c)(3) not-for-profit organization for the future clinic named Trinity Family Health Center and she was starting to raise funds.

Claudette needed a physician on her team, so she turned to her long-time friend and fellow church member, Dr. Deborah Hunter-Brown. Deborah went to medical school and then did her medical residency at Bronx-Lebanon Hospital Center, after which she was in private practice for twenty-two years. During those years she married another physician and they had kids together. But her children were now grown, and she was searching for what God was calling her to do.

When Claudette approached her to be a physician at Trinity, Deborah immediately said, "Your talking to me is not an accident." She too felt prepared for the moment. They met for lunch and began planning the future of the clinic. Claudette's experience as an administrator and Deborah's as a physician made for a strong start to providing compassionate care in the heart of the Bronx. They are clear what God has called them to do, and they are following that calling.

These two stories from Mississippi and New York are from communities that have little in common except they both have great poverty and people who are serious about their faith. What they have seen is that actively caring for the health needs of the community is a way to say "Yes" to what God asks of them, and in the experience of following God's call, they find themselves closer to God—bound to Jesus.

Here's one more story—an enduring one with an inspiring point.

Bob and Will Lightfoot were known around Mobile, Alabama, as "the praying doctors." They had grown up in Montgomery, Alabama, as fourth-generation physicians. Their father, grandfather, and great-grandfather delivered babies, fixed fractures, and took out gallbladders. Will was the older brother and opened a surgery practice in Mobile and offered Bob a deal he couldn't refuse. Together they did the gamut of general surgery.

They kept a "prayer board" in the waiting room where patients would list their prayer requests. It turns out they never got turned down if they asked to pray with someone before a surgery. Bob feels that patients thought, If you are going to operate on me and you have the Lord on your side, then things are probably going to turn out okay.

Bob would have worked his whole career as a surgeon except that in March 1998, he went on a mission trip to Venezuela. As he remembers it, "We were in the middle of nowhere. We slept in hammocks and ate unbelievable food. Our team saw over three thousand patients in four-and-a-half days." They were ten miles from the Colombia border doing all sorts of general medicine when Bob thought, I'm really comfortable doing this, and I think the Lord wants me to be doing something like this in Mobile.

When he returned home to Mobile, as he recalls, "A lady in our church heard us talk about what happened in Venezuela and told me about Medical Outreach Montgomery, which was patterned after Church Health in Memphis. We went to Memphis, where we spent two days in the replication seminar. What had been a fuzzy TV picture all of a sudden got clearer."

"Being in Memphis," Bob said, "let me know that this is what we were supposed to do."

It took three years to get their clinic open. They named it Victory Health Partners. For Bob, the idea of Victory is the most important part. If God is in charge, then victory is certain. The idea of partners is also critical. It has to be a partnership of the health community and the faith community.

By using the Church Health model, Bob and his wife, Tammy, who is a nurse, focused on the uninsured and recruited volunteers of every ilk. While people pushed them to become a FQHC to have a secure funding base, Bob and Tammy responded, "That isn't what God called us to do. We focus on low-income uninsured patients. We are good at staying in our lane. We do the work without relying on government funding and it allows us to do what we believe God expects of us."

Bob left his private practice as a surgeon at the end of 2002 to open Victory Health Partners. Surgeons don't just leave the operating room to start treating hypertension and diabetes. As Bob said, "Surgeons have a different mindset: fix it and move on. If you see a patient three times, that's about it." Bob was now committing himself to forming long-term relationships with patients. It was a little daunting—not to mention all that was required to start the clinic.

To start with, they needed a building. They looked at a lot of buildings. Two were offered for free, but Bob is quick to say they were horrible. And then an eleven-thousand-square-foot building came before them. A hospital owned the building but wanted $850,000. Victory Partners didn't have money like that. They began to pray—just as you would expect from the praying doctors. "We prayed for two years," Bob said. "We spoke to everyone who would listen. And then a gentleman who had done lots of philanthropic things wanted to meet with us. He caught the vision."

With his help the hospital board voted to lease the building to Victory Health Partners for one dollar a year. The building still needed to be renovated, but with the help of volunteers, $75,000 worth of work cost only $5,000. Bob and Tammy, working together, moved things along. A family would paint a room together and do it in memory of someone they loved. Every room had a testimony. The donations flowed to fill up the space.

In 2004 Bob invited me to be the speaker for their first fundraising banquet. I had never been to Mobile. When I got there, it was clear that my only role was to hold up the remarkable work that Bob and Tammy and the rest of their team had accomplished.

By 2021 they had grown to fourteen full-time employees caring for twenty-five thousand patients. They had sixty thousand volunteer hours with a budget of $1.4 million. They also offer counseling, dental care, gynecology, urology, and neurology.

They also addressed the issue of acquiring pharmaceuticals for patients by having a dispensary. This doesn't require having a pharmacist to dispense medicine. Victory Health Partners' sample closet extends to four rooms. They also take full advantage of patient assistance programs, guiding patients to maximum benefit under manufacture programs. With this mix of methods, in 2020 Victory Health Partners provided $42 million worth of pharmaceuticals at no cost to patients. That's a lot of pills.

People in Mobile and in Victory Health Partners refer to Bob as "Doc." It has been twenty years since he was in an operating room. He has become comfortable practicing as a family doctor and has grown into his role as a fundraiser. By the end of 2021, the growth of the program meant they needed a larger building. Doc is up to the task.

Bob said, "We had lots of people say to us 'you are very nice people and that's a nice idea, but it will never work.'" Yet twenty years later, Victory Health Partners is still serving and growing.

Bob believes that when you feel God has called you to do something, there is a sense of the impossible. "We must lay down our impossibility and God can make it possible." It would appear that the success of Victory Health Partners is proof of his belief.

I like the story of Victory Health Partners because it grew out of our early days of offering replication seminars and its success still impresses me. The story illustrates exactly what we hope will happen with all the clinics we work with through the ministry partnership we have now with ECHO. The need remains vast for people to catch the vision of what they can do in their own communities by laying down impossibility and seeing God make it possible.

Faithful Even in Complexity

In reflecting on the role of health care for the church, John Wesley believed that every Methodist Society, and indeed every church, should be involved hands-on in health care. For Wesley, this mostly had to do with the coal miners of western England, but as the Methodist movement traveled to the United States, so did Wesley's view of health and its role in faith communities. In early US history, not everyone was a coal miner, and our communities certainly are made up of many different people now. But they still need health care, and it is still our calling to provide it—even if we are not all Methodists.

John Wesley believed this, and the authors of the New Testament believed that it was a critical link to following Jesus. The complexity of the US health-care system is not a reason for faithful people to step away from the obligation to care for the poor who are sick. Government programs, even the best, are not a substitute for healing ministry under the umbrella of the church. Jesus said, "You always have the poor with you" (Mark 14:7). So far, he has been right. But he went on to say, "and you can show kindness to them whenever you wish." The presence of those in need is not an excuse *not* to help but an ongoing opportunity for generosity. Jesus's call to discipleship clearly requires his followers to be fully engaged in ministries of healing the whole lives, body and spirit, of those we serve.

Whatever form a healing ministry takes in your setting—in your life or your congregation—the right thing is always following Jesus down the path he sets before us.

For Reflection

1. Have you ever not sought care for a medical need because you felt that you couldn't afford the cost? If so, how did that make you feel about your illness, whether small or large, at the time?

2. In reading the brief historical survey of how insurance and safety nets came to be, what new information did you learn?

3. Which of the featured stories in this chapter inspired you most? Why?

TEN

A VISION OF GOD'S REDEMPTION

It seems to me that redemption is the primary purpose of all that we do.

From the moment of our births, we experience being separated from God and we begin a never-ending search to be reconnected. Our actions, our prayers, our longings, our theological musings are all directed toward our hoping to experience being bound tightly to God as we were meant to be.

Jesus's incarnation reveals to us that our bodies are an intricate part of how we fully know God. Our physicality is intrinsically connected to our spiritual life. They are bound together inextricably, and each informs the other as we pursue our quest for redemption throughout life. Much of modern Christianity has been a purely intellectual challenge, and when we are lost in our thinking, we feel alienated from God. When we forget our bodies, we miss that our flesh-and-blood experience can lead us to the connection we seek.

This is why Jesus spent so much of his time as a healer. When our bodies are made whole, the path to God becomes clearer even when we don't know with certainty whether we are spiritually on the right path. Healing the body is a path to wholeness and restoration.

Jesus was constantly aware of the physical experiences of our bodies. He walked everywhere, he constantly connected to people over meals, he wept over those he loved who died. And this was why his death on the cross was so painful. The loss of his body leads him to cry out that God has forsaken him. Our bodies and the care and nurture of them matters to our relationship with God. It is also why, as a physician, I feel the privilege of engaging in patients' lives on both the physical and spiritual level.

I have never felt this more than in my relationship with Ora Alexander.

Ora would never talk about redemption. She would instead insist, "I want you to be filled with the Holy Ghost."

I first met Ora in 1989. I opened the exam-room door and she sat in the chair with her pocketbook on her lap. She was in her late fifties, with long, straight autumn hair. In retrospect I suspect it was a wig, but I'm not good at deciding things like that. She had a very broad smile, with ill-fitting dentures. Through her wire-rimmed glasses, she looked me straight in the eyes.

I went through my routine of questions to figure out why she was there.

"My boss lady said I should come," she said.

With a few more questions, I decided she had hypertension and diabetes that weren't being treated. That was right down my alley.

After a few more minutes, I could tell she was getting tired of all my questions. "Are you done yet?" She sounded irritated.

"Yes, ma'am."

"Good," she said. "Do you want a blessing?"

How do you answer that question other than, "Sure, I'd love a blessing"? Honestly, I had no idea what I was in for.

Ora reached down into her pocketbook and quickly pulled out a small vial of liquid. She shook it and started talking.

"My daughter Michelle is a judge and took me to the Holy Land. We saw all the places in the Bible, and I was touched everywhere we went by the Holy Ghost. I got rebaptized in the Jordan River, and it was just like Jesus reached down and touched me on the head. I was able to bring back a bottle of water from the Jordan. I mixed it with olive oil."

As Ora talked, she stood up. I continued to sit on my stool like I always did. Before I knew it, Ora was lurching above my head with both of her hands on my forehead. It was crystal clear I was no longer in control. She continued to talk while she poured a small amount of liquid into her hand and then pressed deeply into my scalp to make the sign of the cross as she prayed.

"May the power of the Holy Ghost be with you and remain with you."

I wasn't sure what to do, but I closed my eyes and gave myself over to Ora.

She then told me in no uncertain terms, "Stick your hands out."

"Yes, ma'am." What else could I say?

I turned both of my palms upward toward her. She reached again for her holy water. This time she was gentler as she made the sign of the cross on both of my hands and prayed, "May the power of the Holy Ghost be with you as you touch other people as you go through your day. Amen."

I reluctantly pulled my hands back. That was my first of dozens of blessings from Ora. It was a transcendent experience.

Ora was born in 1937 in Selmer, Tennessee, a small town on the edge of the Mississippi Delta. Both of her parents were farmers, which meant that Ora and her eight siblings all had the job of picking cotton. According to Ora, "My daddy could pick three hundred pounds a day and so could I. I could pick more cotton than any boy." For a day's labor she would get paid $1.25. That's it.

"I had sort of a tough streak in me," she said—and I believed it. "I liked to fight. I hit my cousin once in the head, and he thought he was hit with a frying pan." She went on, "And if anyone called me the N-word"—only she said it—"I would bust them in the face. I did that a lot."

I guess that was before she was filled with the Holy Ghost.

In 1953, when Ora was twenty years old, she married a man who soon joined the service. He then left her, and she never heard from him again. Two years later she remarried. With him she had two children and they moved to Memphis. He worked construction until he died in 1983.

Along the way, she started working for the Cannon family. She would work for them for forty-seven years. They were the ones who sent her my way.

It wasn't until 1979 that Ora got religion. She started regularly watching a TV evangelist.

"I sat in my living room and saw him speaking to God. Then one day I was filled with the Holy Ghost and started speaking in tongues."

As she told me this, I interrupted her. "Ora, you were converted and filled with the Holy Spirit and started speaking in tongues while you were alone in your living room?"

She didn't chastise me for my skepticism but recognized a teaching moment. "God can use anything to claim us for his own. I have been living holy ever since. There was a change in my life."

I had to keep pressing. "Ora, what does it mean to live holy?"

"Well, I stopped smoking, started going to church and doing all that the Holy Ghost taught me to do to live holy. It's what happens when Jesus Christ lives in your life. I've been doing it for forty-one years."

She went on, "I had so many things wrong, but God made them all right. And he blessed me with two things—a good mind and a voice to sing. It has made it so that I love being me."

I had no doubt that she did.

Over the years I felt a jump of excitement whenever I saw Ora's name on the patient schedule. It meant I would be getting a blessing. At every visit she would bless my head and my hands with her holy oil. Over time, I depended on her to bless not only me but at least one of our staff members. On more than one occasion, I would find someone I thought could use a blessing and bring the person to the room where I was seeing Ora. I would open the door and say, "This is Ora." Then I would close the door, leaving the person alone with Ora and the Holy Ghost. When the person came out, I didn't really have to say anything. I knew that through Ora, the Holy Ghost was working, even if I didn't fully understand what that means. The Holy Ghost is hard to explain.

At one point, Ora got word that I, from time to time, make my friends a coconut cake. At one of her visits, she said, "My birthday is coming up, and I want you to make me a coconut cake. Will you do that?" There was no saying no. In fact, it felt like an honor.

On Ora's birthday, my wife, Mary, and I carefully wrapped the cake and headed to her house. I had never thought much about where she lived. Her address was on Tillman. I immediately knew what that meant. Ora lived in the Binghampton neighborhood. Although today the neighborhood has had much community revitalization, when Ora moved there it was one of the most dangerous places you could live in Memphis. It was a place of much violence, and it would have been a challenge to be a single woman.

Then again, I was forgetting Ora's proficiency with holding her own in any kind of fight.

It was years later that I better understood how Ora had thrived in Binghampton. It was all about how she understood her community. She told me, "When someone needs help, you help. That's what being a neighbor is." And that is how she lived all her years in her home.

On the day of the cake delivery, we drove up to Ora's house, which sat on a small hill. It was a one-story bungalow with a gated fence around it. We walked up the stairs and rang the doorbell. Ora was there waiting for us. You would have thought I was the king of Siam coming to call on her. With her broad smile and exuberance, she gave first me and then Mary a bear hug before offering us something to drink.

When we said, "No, thank you," Ora's mood changed.

"No one comes to my house without a drink of some sort."

We both then asked for a Coke and sat down on her living room couch. We were in front of the TV where Ora had first been filled with the Holy Ghost.

As though she wasn't expecting it, she exclaimed, "Can you believe that my doctor made me a coconut cake? They told me you wouldn't do it, but I knew you would."

I felt like her gratitude was all I would ever need.

We talked—at least Ora talked, and Mary joined in for a few minutes—but I was out of my element and didn't know what to say. It was hard not being the one in charge of the situation.

For years after, Ora would remind me that I made her a cake on her birthday. It was the most important moment that made us not just doctor and patient but two children of God both trying to find our way back to God.

Redemption. Being filled with the Holy Ghost.

On September 25, 2019, Ora and I sat down together in a StoryCorps booth. StoryCorps has been around for years collecting interviews of people's lives that are then catalogued in the Library of Congress. Their Winnebago van spent a week in Memphis, and someone had the idea that Ora and I should have a conversation with each other, which we both agreed to do. At the time, she was eighty-four years old and I was sixty-five. I had been her doctor for thirty years, but on that day we were connected by a bond that is hard to describe. Its essence is what I have been trying to describe in this book as what healing is. I had tried my best to control her diabetes and her hypertension. At the time, she had a cancer that would take her life within a year. But on that day, our time together was defined by laughter. She summed up our relationship by saying, "I don't think you have ever met anyone like me."

This was certainly true. In the middle of the discussion, she broke out in song. At eighty-four, her voice cracked, but the power of her spirit was so fully alive. At the end of the discussion, I asked how she had come to see what it means to be filled with the Holy Ghost. She replied, "Love everybody. When God blesses me, I bless someone else. The more you give the more you get back."

Ora loved me, and I loved her. And we told each other so in that Story-Corps booth.

That was the last time I saw Ora. She was dying from cancer, but the essence of being alive was fully evident, and her years of both blessing me and showing me a way to "live holy" have stayed with me in deep and profound ways. For three decades—most of my journey so far leading the ministry of Church Health providing quality health care to low-wage uninsured workers—Ora has been evening the playing field between us. When I thought she needed me to take care of her, she showed me that I needed her to take care of me. I knew some things about her physical diseases, but she knew some things about my spiritual yearnings. When she found out I made cakes for my friends, she did not shy away from counting herself as a friend for whom I would make a cake. We lived and grew together in God's redeeming love.

Now every time I make a coconut cake, I remember what Ora said when I asked her if it was any good. With a big broad grin, with a twinkle in her eyes, she told me with jubilation, "It was delicious."

Mercy and Our Neighbors

Jesus's disciples knew body and spirit have something to do with each other, but they didn't always get the relationship right. One time, they saw a man who had been born blind, and they asked Jesus, "Who sinned, this man or his parents?" (John 9:2). They were sure the man was physically blind because of a spiritual offense against God. Jesus's answer was that nobody's sin caused the blindness. Then Jesus spat in the dirt, mixed up some mud, smeared it on the man's eyes, and told him to go wash his face. After the man washed, he could see.

This stirred up quite a bit of controversy. Neighbors tried to convince themselves the man wasn't the same guy they walked past every day. Religious leaders refused to believe his story and threw him out, still not believing someone who sinned as much as he had could be healed—not the most merciful mindset!

This story in John 9 is more about spiritual blindness than physical blindness. The religious leaders refused to open their eyes and see the truth—that God, who is merciful, was at work. Jesus cared enough about the man's blindness to do something about it, and in the process, he pointed to the power of God in the man's life. Jesus said, "Blessed are the merciful, for they will receive mercy" (Matthew 5:7). Our actions should reflect God and the relationship we have with God because we experience God's mercy. And what is mercy but compassion in action?

Jesus was willing to care for Peter's mother-in-law when she was lying in bed with a fever. What a great thing to do for your friend.

A Roman military officer came to Jesus and asked for help for his servant who was suffering with a serious illness. Jesus embraced the need of the servant—and the officer's respect for Jesus's authority—and healed the servant.

When an expert in the Jewish law tried to entice Jesus into debate, Jesus pointed him back to the law the man already knew: love God, love your neighbor. But the expert in the law did what experts do and looked for the loophole. "Who is my neighbor?" In other words, "Who do I really have to be responsible for? And who can I just ignore?"

At this point, Jesus changed the tone of the debate and told a story. A man traveling on the steep and dangerous road between Jerusalem and Jericho fell into the hands of bandits who beat him senseless and left him to die. Religious leaders followed the letter of the law, and rather than risk being temporarily "unclean" by touching a body that might be dead, they crossed to the other side of the road. The traveler who eventually stopped was a Samaritan. The Jews and the Samaritans had nothing good to say about each other and generally went out of their way to avoid one another. Yet this was the traveler who stopped, inconvenienced himself, spent money, and made a commitment to restore health to the Jewish traveler. "Who was the neighbor?" Jesus asked.

The answer was obvious, even to the expert.

Our neighbors are all around us.

The call to mercy is not to figure out the reasonable limits of mercy, but to embrace its unlimited nature. Jesus tells us to put compassion in action, even if it costs us something.

God's mercy for us is unlimited. God poured out rich mercy in sending Jesus to share our flesh. God poured out rich mercy in giving the Holy Spirit to keep us connected to God. When we least deserve it, God pours out mercy on us out of love for us. Jesus gave us enough examples of mercy—compassion in action—to challenge us for a lifetime. Mercy springs up throughout the New Testament, bursting into view just when we think we are free of its demands. Churches face the question of what a healing ministry looks like and come up with answers that fit their situations. It might be a free monthly medical clinic during which Sunday school rooms transform into exam rooms and the fellowship hall is a waiting room. It might be congregations banding together to offer a children's wellness clinic before the start of each school year and giving kids shots, screenings, and school supplies. It might be commitment to regular, budgeted financial and volunteer support at a community clinic that touches the lives of people who would never come through a church door. It might be a faith community nurse who makes herself available to people in the congregation for questions in times of wellness and a comforting presence in times of illness.

Righteousness like a Mighty Stream

I came to Memphis thirty-five years ago because I read somewhere that it was the poorest city in the United States. It did not take long to discover that this was true. But along with economic and health-care injustice, I found vibrant churches across the denominations, neighborhoods with strong identities, and a climate of looking for ways to work together toward healing the scars of the city. As the site of some of the passionate efforts for justice by Martin Luther King Jr., Memphis had a legacy.

Memphis is also the place of King's death.

Countless visitors have stood below the motel balcony where King died and soaked up a sense of the sacred mingled with the history of our country. School children across the land learn to associate "I have a dream" with Martin Luther King Jr. For many of us, those four simple words conjure something big, very big, that is still changing the United States more than five decades later.

Before Martin Luther King Jr. was the iconic leader of the civil rights movement, he was a Baptist preacher and the son of a preacher. He knew the Bible, and he dug past the surface to the heart of God. The cause of justice is the cause of God.

In his famous speech, King said, "No, no, we are not satisfied and we will not be satisfied until justice rolls down like water and righteousness like a mighty stream." He lifted these words from the Old Testament prophet Amos (5:24). Amos was a shepherd who lived during a time of military peace, but a time rife with social injustice.

Oppression of the poor.

A privileged class.

Dishonesty.

Prejudice.

Amos answered the call of God to speak out against injustice to a hostile audience.

Is it any wonder that Martin Luther King Jr. should quote Amos?

Later in the landmark speech, King also quoted the prophet Isaiah and the promise that in preparation for the coming of God, every valley will be lifted up, and the uneven road will be leveled. King dreamed of this vision of justice that Isaiah cast before all our eyes (Isaiah 40:4–5).

And he dreamed that the glory of the Lord would be revealed, and all flesh would see it together.

Together.

"We cannot walk alone," King said about the journey into justice.

By God's grace and with God's help, we still journey together toward the glory of God. The work of making sure the underinsured have equitable access to health care is a journey into justice every day. Every congregation that commits to being a place and agent of healing helps to level the road for the coming of God into someone's life. Every individual who chooses justice becomes part of those rolling, mighty waters.

For Reflection

1. Have you ever met anyone whom Ora reminds you of? What was your encounter or relationship like with the person? In what ways is the person you're thinking of similar to Ora?

2. The author describes the shift that occurred almost immediately in his relationship with Ora because of her initiative. He was not the White,

male, affluent doctor with power to help the Black, female, poor patient. Ora's spiritual gift of anointing him made their shared humanity the central trait of how they interacted. What experience have you had in your own life of an unexpected "equalizing" of a relationship? How did this change you for the better?

3. How would you describe an experience of mercy in your own life, and how did the experience help you have a wider vision of God's redeeming justice?

GROUP DISCUSSION GUIDE

Chapter 1. Living Water in Cactus, Texas

1. On a church mission trip, nurses invited Stephanie Diehlmann to help with a simple task at a makeshift clinic, and the experience set her on a life-changing path. What does this tell us about the church's role in exposing young people to experiences that might shape their callings?

2. Steph Diehlmann and the author are both doctors who opened medical clinics to serve people without access to health care. What do you think their message together might be to people who are *not* doctors?

3. George is one of the Lost Boys from Sudan, where the civil war traumatized his life—perhaps permanently. How does his story help us as people of faith reflect on what it means to help people have access to health care? What does it mean for someone in George's shoes to be healthy?

4. Cactus, Texas, is a meatpacking town. Most of us take for granted that we can go to the store and pick up cuts of meat and take them home and never think much about how they got there. How can the picture in this chapter of Cactus, the people who live there, and their needs, make us more attuned to the nature of communities other than our own?

5. What lessons might we in the twenty-first century embrace more deeply about what Jesus, God's own Son, shows us about health?

6. The author says, "Jesus cared about bodies because he cared about the whole person in relationship to God." What does a life of faith in the body mean to you?

7. The author reminds us of the tradition of healing ministry in the early church. Because of this, the Romans asked, "Who is your God that I might worship him?" What can we learn from this that applies to health ministry in our century?

Chapter 2. Flipping between a Living and Health Care

1. The author admits he took visitors to Beale Street to see the flippers for entertainment and passed by the buckets they used in order to make a living, essentially seeing them for his own purposes and not as true persons, until the first flipper turned up in his exam room. What experience in your life has helped change the way you view people who are different from you?

2. The author wanted to help Lillian because her need was genuine and because she was caught up in a dysfunctional system that offered her no practical solutions. But he also acknowledges a measure of guilt that his own organization's guidelines had failed her once before. In what ways can guilt function positively to motivate us to step up to help those in need? Or do you dispute this motivation?

3. "The Gradys" is a hospital that bears in its history a story of racial injustice, and in its shadows, Good Samaritan Health Clinic is still serving people of color who unjustly have less access to care a century later. How does this story make us think about the stories built into the histories of our own communities that we need to hear and address?

4. Good Samaritan Health Clinic is similar in mission and ministry to the author's own ministry at Church Health. Can you think of ministries in your own community that offer health care for uninsured individuals that you perhaps haven't thought much about in the past?

5. Toward the end of the chapter, the author lists some general ideas for how people who are not physicians can get involved in health-care ministry. What other ideas can you think of to add to this list?

6. The unbelieving Roman emperor Julian wrote, "Now we can see what it is that makes those Christians such powerful enemies of our gods. It is the brotherly love which they manifest toward the sick and poor, the thoughtful manner in which they care for the dead, and the purity of their own lives." He compared the Christian practices against the

practices of those who followed Roman gods. If you were writing this comparison for readers today, how would you reword it? Do you think people perceive Christians today as distinctive in their care for the sick?

7. Early Christians formed a community to be God's active healing presence in the world. What two or three concepts do you think are essential for Christians today to grab hold of to see being an active healing presence as part of their identity?

Chapter 3. Faith during a Pandemic

1. Sometimes when we face someone else's illness, our first instinct is to guard our own welfare. Do you think this is a legitimate response or one we need to learn to temper?

2. How might facing personal loss affect our perspectives on others who face loss, particularly in times like a pandemic when many people may be suffering illness, financial devastation, and death?

3. What were some of the brightest and most inspiring ways you saw people of faith responding during the COVID-19 pandemic?

4. What were some of the most perturbing ways you saw people of faith responding during the COVID-19 pandemic? What do you think makes the difference between these actions and the inspiring choices of others?

5. The author says that in light of the needs and inequities the COVID-19 pandemic has revealed, "Re-embracing the healing ministry of the church is one of the great opportunities we now have before us." Do you agree or disagree? Why?

6. Name some specific ways people of faith can move forward with a broader view of equity in health care in your own community because the pandemic taught them lessons they didn't expect.

7. In what ways are healing and hope fundamentally connected? Can you give some examples of how you've seen this connection in action?

Chapter 4. Why Do Those Pills Cost So Much?

1. This chapter tells the story of several patients whose diagnoses ranged from something simple to complex combinations of chronic diseases. None of them could afford the medications that would make their lives

comfortable in the long term. How do you respond to the composite picture of life without needed medications that these stories of real people create?

2. Developing, manufacturing, and selling pharmaceuticals is an industry that runs on profit. On the one hand, it's reasonable for people to earn a living. On the other hand, it's unreasonable that people can't afford basic medications. As people of faith, what principles can we use to reconcile these two truths?

3. Often stories about the cost of life-saving drugs such as insulin make the news with the face of someone for whom the struggle to pay for medications is all-consuming even as prices rise. Sometimes the story has a sad ending. Sometimes the story points to assistance programs, but they are difficult to navigate and less than ideal. What principles of justice could we be using as a lens as we seek solutions to the cost of medications for people who need them but can't afford them?

4. In what ways are well-insured people often separated from the true cost of medications? When you fill a prescription with insurance, do you ever look at the amount you "saved" by having insurance? How do you respond emotionally and intellectually?

5. How might the safety net of health insurance keep us from confronting the need to advocate for access to medications for those without insurance? How might the experience of being insured be a motivator to advocate for affordable medications?

6. This chapter contains a section about the author's own efforts to supply common maintenance medications to his patients, which took significant energy and innovation. What lessons can we take from this example to apply in our community even if the form of the solution is different than what the author tried in his setting?

7. The author makes the point that the early church organized itself to care for the daily needs of the people. In what ways can we apply this principle to addressing affordable medications?

Chapter 5. Back to Work with Duct-Taped Knees and Broken Smiles

1. Melvin "Too Tall" Moore's story is both heartfelt and heart-aching. In a situation like this, it can be hard to know how to begin to respond. How

do you find yourself reacting when you read about—or even more, meet someone—whose story is so complex? How do we find and offer hope in situations that are likely far outside our own experiences?

2. Paul is one example of someone whose social circumstances led to what seems obvious to people like Paul—keep putting off his own care so he can keep looking after his family. What personal experiences do you have that help you understand Paul's situation? How would you define doing our best for one another in circumstances like these?

3. When we read Jorge's story, we probably all feel like a child his age should not have to face that much serious dental work, nor should he have to be aware of the financial stress that treatment can cause for his family. What did you learn from Jorge's story that you didn't know about how dental health intersects with poverty, low-income wages, or lack of insurance? What thoughts do you have about how your own community can respond compassionately and effectively to these issues?

4. Brett and Angela Bymaster moved to an underserved neighborhood in San Jose, California, and joined a church with a vision and have remained in the same community for the long haul. This has allowed them to know how the resources and networks can be leveraged to serve those in greatest need and also to respond with personal care because they've nurtured relationships with people they've cared for. What resources and networks are available in your local community that are being, or could be, leveraged to address obstacles to health care that arise from social and economic circumstance?

5. Review some of the healing miracles in the book of Acts mentioned in this chapter. In what ways do these stories inspire us to engage in ministries of wellness for both body and spirit?

6. The author says, "Healing that flows from personal care, preventive activities, medical methods, and technology announces that the kingdom of God is here." Describe some practical ways the church shows the here-and-now nature of the kingdom of God through health and healing activities congregations can participate in.

7. Social issues can be complex, and how we posture to respond can be divisive. What attitudes and priorities can we hold onto tightly to respond faithfully to the calling God gives us, and which should we hold more loosely? How do we choose which we put in each column?

Chapter 6. No Papers, No Health Care

1. When Maria first came to Church Health's clinic, trust threatened to interfere with the care she needed. Can you think of ways lack of trust in your own life, or the lives of people you've known personally, has interfered with receiving needed health care?

2. Because the author established trust with Maria in smaller matters, she returned confidently in larger matters, even though she was undocumented. Why is trust especially important in this scenario?

3. Wendy's trauma was the reason she left her home and almost didn't make it to the United States safely, and Maria experienced injury in coming to her assistance. How does hearing personal stories like these help us understand that issues may be more complex than we realize?

4. Before beginning to read about the life work of Janelle Goetcheus among housing-insecure people, how aware were you that even US citizens might be unable to properly establish their identities to access resources they are entitled to? Have you ever had to replace an important identity document? How did the experience shed light on what the experience might be like if you had to start from scratch with no other corroborating documents?

5. Perhaps you are reading this book because you are wondering about your own sense of calling to be more deeply engaged with some form of ministry for health equity. What reflections do you have about the concept of "the called" after reading this chapter?

6. Read Matthew 25:31–46. What part of this passage inspires you the most? What part challenges you the most? Why?

7. Janelle Goetcheus's experience at Church of the Saviour is one of finding and forming mission in small community. What do you think would be the nature of a community that discerned a mission together?

Chapter 7. Tackling Preventable Chronic Disease

1. What do you think of the very direct approach the author took with Roger in the beginning, to the point of making him defensive and angry? Would you normally advise this as a path toward healing? Why or why not?

2.   The author makes the case that many people with chronic diseases, even those who may have been prescribed medications to control them, still don't understand the dangers of the diseases and why it's important to comply with medical advice. What are your thoughts about people's attitudes toward taking medications—or not taking them—when their health is at risk?

3.   The author also makes the case that in many situations, the rampant chronic diseases that plague our society right now, especially type 2 diabetes, hypertension, and heart disease, are preventable or manageable with lifestyle changes rather than pharmaceuticals (though sometimes both are needed). How do you perceive the prevailing attitudes toward lifestyle issues that are linked to increasing occurrence of these chronic diseases? Can the ship be turned? What would it take for success?

4.   The Open Arms clinic in Arlington, Texas, started to see dramatic improvements when they began expecting more from their patients. How can more medical providers strike the right tone of expressing that they genuinely care about the welfare of patients without giving patients a free pass about what they can do to help their own health?

5.   Heal the City in Amarillo, Texas, also tackled chronic diseases by both focusing on the whole person and expecting patients to participate in making changes to improve their health. Most health clinics cannot be as overtly faith-based as Open Arms and Heal the City are—but churches can be. In what ways can your church step up its game in helping people be accountable for daily choices that contribute to the level of health they experience?

6.   The author argues that we don't have the balance right between what we expect from technology in preventive health care and appreciating the gifts of God in bountiful varieties of food and the ways our bodies were created to work. What do you think stands in the way for most people of moving toward healthier ownership of what they can do for themselves to pursue healthy living? How can we help one another past these obstacles?

7.   In response to the woman who had been ill for twelve years, Jesus said, "Daughter, your faith has made you well; go in peace, and be healed of your disease" (Mark 5:34). Explain in your own words how you understand the relationship between faith and health. How does this apply to the area of preventing or managing chronic diseases?

Chapter 8. What's on Your Mind Is in Your Body

1. What was the most gripping part of Zyanya's story for you? In what ways did it bring into focus that we cannot separate the health of our minds from the health of our bodies?

2. Unfortunately, Zyanya did not get the best advice from her pastor after she finally had the courage to tell him what happened. What do you think are the strengths and weaknesses of the way people in churches respond to others who have been wounded in traumatic situations?

3. The author says, "Half of the people who come to primary care doctors like me have no physical medical problem. They are there because of their mental and emotional health needs. These days, people come to the doctor for reasons they used to visit the priest or pastor. Why is that? It is partly because people have decreased trust in the clergy and partly because clergy are less well trained or available to deal with matters of the heart. Unfortunately, physicians are equally ill-equipped to care for matters of the spirit." What do you think causes decrease in trust in the clergy—or even the wider church—when it comes to mental and emotional health needs? What would it take for churches to do a better job and regain trust?

4. Many people in the church, and in the culture as a whole, are uncomfortable around issues related to mental health or behavioral health, such as addiction issues. In what ways might better understanding of our creation as body and spirit that cannot be separated be used in local congregations to make talking about mental health safer without fear of stigma?

5. Bishop Young had a galvanizing experience about mental health in the church. Sadly, it was tragic. What practical lessons can local congregations take from that story that can lead to being proactive about mental health in the church?

6. Matt Russell had a different type of galvanizing experience about mental health in the church. How can you reflect on the failures of the traditional church to respond to mental health in redeeming ways? What theological reflections might you apply to make people's experience more positive in your own congregational settings?

7. The author points out that in Luke 10, Jesus's followers went out in part-

nership and were astonished at what became of their ministry. Even if a church regains trust as a safe place to talk about mental health, there will always be a place for medical professionals. Based on what you know about health systems in your community, what steps could a local church take to make sure it has appropriate partnerships with medical professionals to turn to when needed?

Chapter 9. Echoes of God's Love

1. What has been your own story of being insured or uninsured? Good insurance or not so good? Needing it or hardly using it? How does your personal story shape your feelings about US health care?

2. When you read the historical survey section of this chapter covering how private and public insurance emerged, in what ways do you see the church finding or losing its way in caring for those in need?

3. As we have seen in earlier chapters of this book and in this chapter, many of the reasons people don't have access to a system that depends on health insurance are complicated. Against this backdrop, how would you describe how people of faith should respond?

4. This chapter features several people who got involved in providing health care to people who are underserved. What do they have in common that drives them?

5. Some of the people we read about in this chapter were doctors, but others weren't. Mary Leslie had no health-care background, and Claudette was a dietician turned administrator. What can we learn from this diversity of callings about what it takes to make a difference in health care?

6. In earlier chapters, we encountered other clinics using the Church Health model. In this chapter, we saw more fully the hunger of congregations and communities over the decades to do something like what Church Health has done because the need for health-care access for the uninsured or people with low incomes remains so high. In what ways might catching a vision of this larger movement inspire action at local levels that even government programs won't solve?

7. The author is a Methodist minister, so he mentioned John Wesley, the founder of Methodism, several times in the book. In this chapter he points out that Wesley believed every Christian community should

be involved in hands-on health ministry. How do you respond to this thought? What might that look like in your congregation? If a group were to commit to a health-care ministry of some form, whether or not it was a medical clinic, what might be the next steps to explore?

Chapter 10. A Vision of God's Redemption

1.   This chapter focuses our attention on our longing to connect to God. The author says, "It seems to me that redemption is the primary purpose of all that we do. From the moment of our births, we experience being separated from God and we begin a never-ending search to be reconnected." Overall, how did this final chapter of the book draw you in to this theme of our ultimate healing?

2.   The author says, "Healing the body is a path to wholeness and restoration." Do you agree or disagree? Why or why not?

3.   The author's longtime patient—and friend—Ora features prominently in this chapter. He was eager to share the experience of Ora's blessings with others he thought needed it by putting them in the room with her and then leaving. He says, "Then I would close the door, leaving the person alone with Ora and the Holy Ghost." How do you think you might react if you'd had this experience with Ora?

4.   What is most touching to you about the relationship between the author and Ora? What are the most significant lessons we can learn about healing work from the way their relationship took on an equalized shape very early?

5.   Jesus said, "Blessed are the merciful, for they will receive mercy" (Matthew 5:7). How does our experience of the mercy of God intersect with exploring a calling to care for the underserved neighbors in our community in merciful ways? If we have an insufficient understanding of mercy, how might that color our views of serving those in need?

6.   The author reminds us that the prophet Amos was a shepherd who lived during a time rife with social injustice. One of the most quoted verses from the book of Amos exhorts us to "let justice roll down like waters, and righteousness like an ever-flowing stream" (Amos 5:24). When we think about health justice, as we have throughout this book, what would a vision of an ever-flowing stream of righteousness look like?

7. We hear the words of Isaiah 40:3–5 most often during the seasons of Advent or Christmas. A voice calls out to prepare the way of the Lord, lifting up the valleys and making low the hills and the rough places a plain to reveal the glory of God. How can we take to heart this picture of God's coming redemption in our own journey to level the road of health justice and give those we care for a picture of the glory of God?

ACKNOWLEDGMENTS

Church Health opened its doors on September 1, 1987. Since that day, hundreds if not thousands of people have caught the vision of what the work of health ministry means. My hope is that this book will be a testament to the meaning of this work long after all those who helped start Church Health are gone. When it comes to the writing of this book, I am grateful to all those whose stories I tell and who are working in their own right in health ministries around the country.

There are a few whose support has especially made it possible for this book to exist. First and foremost is Susan Martins Miller, who began writing with me over a decade ago for the book *Health Care You Can Live With*. Since then, she has been a full-time writer for Church Health and edits every word I publish. There is no way this book could have been done without her heavy lifting.

It is also because of Susan that I was introduced to my agent, Rachelle Gardner. The world of publishing is complicated and requires true professionals, which Rachelle certainly is.

Rachel Davis was invaluable in casting the vision for what this book might be.

My executive assistants who helped in a variety of ways include Anna Joy Tamayo, Bryana Polk, and Cynthia Byrd Shaw.

I am thankful for my senior leadership team who pulls the work of Church Health forward. Jenny Bartlett-Prescott, Jennie Robbins, Ann

Langston, Mike Sturdivant, and Lois McFarland are all immensely talented and dedicated to the work we do together. I am thankful to the two chairs of the Church Health board during the time I was writing, Rob Carter and Mike Glenn. Your leadership in our work has been critical at challenging times. We are stronger because of you.

And last, my soul mate is my wife, Mary Gilleland Morris. She helps keep me moving forward and gives me a place to rest. In her I find my spirit renewed.

NOTES

Chapter Two

1. Jennifer Tolbert, Kendal Orgera, and Antony Damico, "Key Facts about the Uninsured Population," Kaiser Family Foundation, November 6, 2020, https://www.kff.org/uninsured/issue-brief/key-facts-about-the-uninsured -population/ (accessed September 21, 2021).

2. Paul Houchens, Dave Liner, Annie Man, Andrew Naugle, Doug Norris, and Scott Weltz, "2021 Milliman Medical Index," Milliman Research Report, May 27, 2021, https://www.milliman.com/en/insight/2021-milliman-medical -index (accessed September 21, 2021).

3. See note 1, above.

4. See note 1, above.

5. The National Association of Free and Charitable Clinics, *2019 Annual Report*, https://www.nafcclinics.org/content/about-us (accessed September 22, 2021).

Chapter Three

1. Maria Elena Martínez, Jesse N. Nodora, and Luis G. Carvajal-Carmona, "The Dual Pandemic of COVID-19 and Systemic Inequities in U.S. Latino Communities," *Cancer* 127, no. 10 (May 15, 2021): 1546–50, https://doi.org/10.1002 /cncr.33401 (accessed September 22, 2021).

2. Samantha Artiga, Bradley Corallo, and Olivia Pham, "Racial Disparities in COVID-19: Key Findings from Available Data and Analysis," Kaiser Family Foundation, August 17, 2020, https://www.kff.org/racial-equity-and-health -policy/issue-brief/racial-disparities-covid-19-key-findings-available-data -analysis/ (accessed September 22, 2021).

3. Brea L. Perry, Brian Aronson, and Bernice A. Pescosolido, "Pandemic Precarity: COVID-19 Is Exposing and Exacerbating Inequalities in the American Heartland," *Proceedings of the National Academy of Sciences* 118, no. 8 (February 2021), https://doi.org/10.1073/pnas.2020685118 (accessed September 21, 2022).

4. Jesse Bradford, Erica Coe, Kana Enomoto, and Matt White, "COVID-19 and Rural Communities: Protecting Rural Lives and Health," McKinsey & Company, March 10, 2021, https://www.mckinsey.com/industries/health care-systems-and-services/our-insights/covid-19-and-rural-communities -protecting-rural-lives-and-health (accessed September 22, 2021).

Chapter Four

1. Robert A. Hegele, "Insulin Affordability," *The Lancet* 5, no. 5 (May 1, 2017): 324, https://doi.org/10.1016/S2213-8587(17)30115-8 (accessed September 29, 2021).

2. Matel Mikulic, "Pharmaceutical Spending Per Capita in Selected Countries as of 2019," Statista, April 15, 2021, https://www.statista.com/statistics /266141/pharmaceutical-spending-per-capita-in-selected-countries/ (accessed September 29, 2021); "Health at a Glance 2019: OECD Indicators," OECD Publishing, Paris, https://doi.org/10.1787/4dd50c09-en (accessed September 29, 2021).

3. Andrew W. Mulcahy, Christopher Whaley, Mahlet G. Rebekka, Daniel Schwam, Nathaniel Edenfield, and Alejandro U. Becerra-Ornelas, "International Prescription Drug Price Comparisons: Current Empirical Estimates and Comparisons with Previous Studies," RAND Corporation, 2020, https:// www.rand.org/pubs/research_reports/RR2956.html (accessed September 29, 2021).

Chapter Five

1. Krutika Amin, Gary Claxton, Giorlando Ramirez, and Cynthia Cox, "How Does Cost Affect Access to Care?" Peterson-KFF Health System Tracker, January 5, 2021, https://www.healthsystemtracker.org/chart-collection/cost -affect-access-care/ (accessed September 27, 2021).

2. "PAI-NORC Survey Shows High Deductible Health Plans Are a Barrier to Needed Care," Physicians Advocacy Institute, http://www.physiciansadvo cacyinstitute.org/Advocacy/Health-Plan-Advocacy/High-Deductible-Health -Plans (accessed September 27, 2021). Links to a PowerPoint and the full study are available at this site as well.

3. Jennifer Tolbert, Kendal Orgera, and Antony Damico, "Key Facts about the Uninsured Population," Kaiser Family Foundation, November 6, 2020, https://www.kff.org/uninsured/issue-brief/key-facts-about-the-uninsured -population/ (accessed September 21, 2021).

4. "Poverty and Health: The Family Medicine Perspective (Position Paper)," American Academy of Family Physicians, https://www.aafp.org/about /policies/all/poverty-health.html (accessed September 27, 2021).

Chapter Six

1. "Immigration," USA Facts, https://usafacts.org/issues/immigration /?utm_source=google&utm_medium=cpc&utm_campaign=ND-Immigration &gclid=CjoKCQjw18WKBhCUARIsAFiW7JxwNvgWSje2vhF6_Jl9Tyh3Nw RMqCDECZWM_KLoNlf-KSOVZbWG-QgaAjbbEALw_wcB (accessed September 27, 2021).

2. Jen Manual Krogstad, Jeffrey S. Passel, and D'Vera Cohn, "5 Facts About Illegal Immigration in the U.S.," Pew Research Center, June 12, 2019, https://www.pewresearch.org/fact-tank/2019/06/12/5-facts-about-illegal -immigration-in-the-u-s/ (accessed September 28, 2021).

3. Jeffrey S. Passel and D'Vera Cohn, "U.S. Unauthorized Immigrant Total Dips to Lowest Level in a Decade," Pew Research Center, November 27, 2018, https://www.pewresearch.org/hispanic/2018/11/27/u-s-unauthorized -immigrant-total-dips-to-lowest-level-in-a-decade/ (accessed September 28, 2021).

4. See note 1, above.

5. Mark Hugo Lopez, Jeffrey S. Passel, and D'Vera Cohn, "Key Facts About the Changing U.S. Unauthorized Immigrant Population," Pew Research Center, April 12, 2021, https://www.pewresearch.org/fact-tank/2021/04/13/key -facts-about-the-changing-u-s-unauthorized-immigrant-population/ (accessed September 28, 2021).

6. Abby Budiman, "Key Findings about U.S. Immigrants," Pew Research Center, August 20, 2020, https://www.pewresearch.org/fact-tank/2020/08/20 /key-findings-about-u-s-immigrants/ (accessed September 28, 2021).

Chapter Seven

1. "About the Center," National Center for Chronic Disease Prevention and Health Promotion at the CDC, https://www.cdc.gov/chronicdisease/center/ (accessed September 30, 2021).

2. Wullianullur Raghupathi and Viju Raghupathi, "An Empirical Study of Chronic Diseases in the United States: A Visual Analytics Approach to Public Health," *Environmental Research and Public Health* 15, no. 3 (March 1, 2018): 431, https://www.ncbi.nlm.nih.gov/pmc/articles/PMC5876976/ (accessed September 30, 2021).

3. Andrea S. Christopher, Danny McCormick, Steffie Woolhandler, David U. Himmelstein, David H. Bor, and Andrew P. Wilper, "Access to Care and Chronic Disease Oucomes among Medicaid-insured Persons Versus the Uninsured," *American Journal of Public Health* 106, no. 1 (January 2016): 63–69, https://ajph.aphapublications.org/doi/10.2105/AJPH.2015.302925 (accessed September 20, 2021).

4. Rachel Garfield, Kendal Orgera, and Anthony Damico, "The Uninsured and the ACA: A Primer—Key Facts about Health Insurance and the Uninsured amidst Changes to the Affordable Care Act," Kaiser Family Foundation, January 25, 2019, https://www.kff.org/uninsured/report /the-uninsured-and-the-aca-a-primer-key-facts-about-health-insurance -and-the-uninsured-amidst-changes-to-the-affordable-care-act/ (accessed September 30, 2019).

5. Reaves Houston, Susan Keen, Chelsea Deitzelzeig, Hannah Jones, Sarah Laible, Catherine Sauter, and Ross J. Simpson, "Abstract P076: Increased Burden of Chronic Illness Among Insured Compared to Uninsured Sudden Death Victims," *Circulation* 143 (May 18, 2021), https://doi.org/10.1161/circ.143.suppl _1.P076 (accessed September 30, 2021).

Chapter Eight

1. "Improving Access to Children's Mental Health Care," Centers for Disease Control and Prevention, https://www.cdc.gov/childrensmentalhealth /access.html (accessed October 1, 2021).

2. Stacy Hodgkinson, Leandra Godoy, Lee Savio Beers, and Amy Lewin, "Improving Mental Mental Health Access for Low-Income Children and Families in the Primary Care Setting," *Pediatrics* 139, no. 1 (January 2017), https://www.ncbi.nlm.nih.gov/pmc/articles/PMC5192088/ (accessed January 20, 2022).

3. "Access to Healthcare and Mental Health Services Is Limited When You Live in Poverty," North Carolina Community Action Association, June 12, 2020, https://www.nccaa.net/post/access-to-healthcare-and-mental-health -services-is-limited-when-you-live-in-poverty (accessed October 1, 2021). See also "New Study Reveals Lack of Access as Root Cause of Mental Health Crisis in America," National Council for Mental Wellbeing, https://www.thenation alcouncil.org/press-releases/new-study-reveals-lack-of-access-as-root-cause -for-mental-health-crisis-in-america/ (accessed October 1, 2021).

4. "2020 Access to Care Data," Mental Health America, https://mhana tional.org/issues/2020/mental-health-america-access-care-data (accessed October 1, 2021).

5. Dhruv Khullar, "The Largest Health Disparity We Don't Talk About: Americans with Serious Mental Illnesses Die 15 to 30 Years Earlier than Those Without," *The New York Times*, May 30, 2018, https://www.nytimes.com/2018 /05/30/upshot/mental-illness-health-disparity-longevity.html (accessed October 1, 2021).

6. Maria Cohut, "Why Mental Healthcare Is Not a Safe Space for Undocumented Migrants," *Medical News Today*, July 14, 2020, https://www.medi calnewstoday.com/articles/why-mental-healthcare-is-not-a-safe-space-for -undocumented-migrants (accessed October 1, 2021). See also Luz M. Garcini, Juan M. Peña, Angela P. Gutierrez, Christopher P. Fagundes, Hector Lemus, Suzanne Lindsay, and Elizabeth A. Klonoff, "One Scar Too Many: The Associations Between Traumatic Events and Psychological Distress Among Undocumented Mexican Immigrants," *Journal of Traumatic Stress* 30, no. 5 (October 27, 2017): 456–62, https://doi.org/10.1002/jts.22216 (accessed October 1, 2021) and Carol Cleaveland and Cara Frankenfeld, "They Kill People Over Nothing: An Exploratory Study of Latina Immigrant Trauma," *Journal of Social Service*

Research 46, no. 4 (2020), https://doi.org/10.1080/01488376.2019.1602100 (accessed October 1, 2021).

Chapter Nine

1. "Health Center Program: Impact and Growth," Health Resources & Services Administration, https://bphc.hrsa.gov/about/healthcenterprogram /index.html (accessed October 6, 2021). See also https://data.hrsa.gov/tools /data-reporting/program-data (accessed October 6, 2021).

2. The National Association of Free & Charitable Clinics, *NAFC Member Data Report 2021*, https://www.nafcclinics.org/content/tools (accessed October 7, 2021).

3. ECHO is a charity and partner ministry of Church Health in Memphis, Tennessee, committed to echoing God's love by aiding the development of charitable clinics, ultimately inspiring faith communities across the United States to establish whole-person health-care ministries for the underserved. For more information visit www.echoclinics.org.